CW00507339

OPTIMAL SEX LIFE

Advance Praise for

OPTIMAL SEX LIFE

~~~~~~~~~~~~~~~~~~~~~~~~~~~~~~~~

"I strongly recommend this book. Aaron shares his unique style of de-armoring that you will not find anywhere else. This book will show you the secrets for to how to open a body, the way Aaron would open mine. Even a practice session with Aaron would leave me in a state of no-mind afterwards: to just be, glow, and buzz with energy from my sex area into my every cell. I felt more feminine, soft, and sensual . . . the sexual me fully alive. It has been a pleasure to be a steady guide and encouragement in his growth as a professional in this field, where trusted, quality, male workers are scarce. I look forward for more in years to come."

—SUSANNE ROURSGAARD, Founder of the Gaia Method

"Aaron's work is outstanding. I have been working and teaching in the field of sacred sexuality and conscious relating for many years. I have received countless sessions and worked with many different people. My nose for quality is top notch, and this is what Aaron is: Top notch. If you EVER get the chance to work with him, GO FOR IT. He's highly skilled, respective, conscious, and his hands are absolutely beyond magic. This book will show you how to do the same."

—SANNA SANITA, Swedens Leading Sacred
Sexuality & Consciousness Teacher

"I get many phone calls but there was something about the authenticity and honesty in Aaron's voice that interested my inner scientist, journalist, and therapist; moreover it whispered to the woman Signe. He had no ambitions, which gave me the unique experience to let go of control and judgement and allowed me to surrender. The experience was intense, very intense . . . a voyage into myself, to encounter any sensations that might arrive. He was like a Sherpa guide. With my own voice and breath, the pain transformed into pleasure. His touch gave me a compass that has set me off on a path to more tangible teaching and giving others this experience. I'm still passing it on, and this book can do the same for you."

—SIGNE BENTZEN, Author, Tantric Sexologist,
and Couples Counsleor

"Aaron is the kind of person you notice right away. He radiates passion, depth, joy, compassion, and love, and so does his work. What differentiates Aaron's techniques from all others that I've tried, is his ability to make you feel so comfortable, safe and loved; while releasing old traumas, shame and tensions. He makes healing pleasurable, simple, and fun! I have tried a lot in this field of work, but I can truly say that I have met no other as warm hearted, skilled, and professional as Aaron. His approach and techniques can forever change your body and your life. I love this book. Aaron takes so much knowledge and makes it come together in way that seems easy and understandable for even newcomers to grasp."

—GRY DAGMAR SCHØDT MØBERG, Tantric Bodyworker,
Shamanistic Therapist, and Leadership Mentor

OPTIMAL
SEX
LIFE

An Exercise Book for
De-Armoring and Tantric Sex

AARON MICHAEL, MA

OPTIMAL SEX LIFE
Copyright © 2018 TRANSFREEMATION IVS

All rights reserved. No part of this book may be reproduced in any manner whatsoever without written permission from the Publisher, except in the case of brief quotations embedded in critical articles and reviews, and certain other noncommercial uses permitted by copyright law.

TRANSFREEMATION IVS
Copenhagen, Denmark
OptimalSexLife.com
contact@optimalsexlife.com
Facebook: facebook.com/OptimalSexLife

ISBN: 978-87-97115-0-5

Cover design by Nis von Steelen
Illustrations by Adam Beker, based on drawings by Aaron Michael
Interior design by www.DominiDragoone.com

9 8 7 6 5 4 3 2

I dedicate this book to all the people who
have supported me along the way and encouraged me to always
go forward and never give up on my dreams, and to my beloved
empress, queen, and muse of my life—my wife, Stine. May I
and the profits of this book forever serve you and our relationship
in alignment with the love and plan of The All. I love you...

DISCLAIMER

All content found in this book, *Optimal Sex Life,* including: text, images, audio, or other formats, was created for informational purposes only. Offerings for continuing education credits are clearly identified and the appropriate target audience is identified. The Content is not intended to be a substitute for professional medical advice, diagnosis, or treatment. Always seek the advice of your physician or other qualified health provider with any questions you may have regarding a medical condition. Never disregard professional medical advice or delay in seeking it because of something you have read in this book or on OptimalSexLife.com.

If you think you may have a medical emergency, call your doctor, go to the emergency department, or call 911 immediately. TRANSFREEMATION IVS does not recommend or endorse any specific tests, physicians, products, procedures, opinions, or other information that may be mentioned in *Optimal Sex Life.* Reliance on any information provided by TRANSFREEMATION IVS, TRANSFREEMATION IVS employees, contracted writers, or medical professionals presenting content for publication to TRANSFREEMATION IVS is solely at your own risk.

CONTENTS

FOREWORD

We all want to gain knowledge and experience results. I do not have a wall full of degrees and a list of titles. I *do* have a BA with Honors in Linguistics from the University of Michigan, Ann Arbor. I also have an Elite MA in Cognitive Semiotics from Aarhus University, Denmark. I wrote my thesis on the psychology and neuroscience of love, and performed conversational analysis of interactions to identify the key elements that spark attraction in courtship. However, I am neither a medical doctor nor a guru. I am but a simple man, which I hope will convince you that anyone is capable of nurturing their optimal sex life with time and dedication.

My education as a sex coach has been heuristic and multifaceted. In each chapter, I give you a bit of my story so you will have "the where, the why, and the what" of each exercise. Feel free to skip "the where" if you are uninterested in knowing where I obtained this knowledge. It is only there for those who are curious.

As for the "why" and the "what," the exercises are numbered and build upon one another. I strongly recommend taking the time to follow them sequentially for best results. The first exercises may seem simple at first, yet their application is the foundation for your practice, success, and enjoyment.

Optimal sex is much less about technique and capabilities, which you will gain in this book, and far more about finding your optimal partner and practice partners. As such, Chapter 7: *Choosing Your Partner(s)*, could have easily been the first chapter. However, the exercises change your physical make-up and align you with yourself, which in turn prepares you for and attracts those best suited for experiencing and nurturing growth with you. For this reason, I have included this chapter towards the end.

As for the exercises, I am building a video library for those who wish to subscribe. Here is the link:

www.aaronmichaelmethod.com/exercises

INTRODUCTION

Take courage and have patience because within this book, you can learn a powerful method for feeling more with every touch, and for guiding others to encounter more pleasure in their own bodies. At first, you may discover that you are experiencing pain and using a lot of effort to lower your psychological defenses before encountering pleasure. Some may call this *de-armoring*. Armor is the overall physical posture and psychological character we adopt to ensure that we contain the emotional and physical pain **and pleasure** which we fear to express or acknowledge. Armor inhibits physical and mental plasticity, which blocks the flow of movement and expressivity of emotional energy throughout the body. Over time, the effect is the closing down and rigidity of our persona and body . . . your expression of self. De-armoring is the technique by which you remove your psychosomatic blocks, release the pain and pleasure you spend so much energy inhibiting, and regain your literal sense of self. The mind and body are one. The result is the freeing up of tremendous amounts of energy that once was used to contain your self, and that now becomes available for you to achieve your goals and realize your dreams. If you contain pain, then it is most often pain you will experience when pain first leaves your body. If it is numbness, then you will often times experience impatience. However, know that whether it is discomfort, pain, or that you literally feel no sensation at all when you or another touches your stomach, caresses your breasts, or attempts to pleasure any other part of you, then it does not have to remain this way. You can have hope that your experience will change!

In fact, you are meant to feel the exact opposite of pain, which is your pleasure—and this you can learn to have. It is your birthright, though you may find yourself resistant to truly feeling into your body's current state of affairs. Accepting touch, and dealing with our psychological, sexual or physical pain can be uncomfortable, and so can "letting go" of this pain or numbness. However, once you let go of trauma on one side of the healing coin, an even greater pleasant surprise will likely await you on the other side, so continue to be patient with yourself as you grow your pleasure. When most people think of fear, we think of pain and fighting, but what I find never ceases to surprise people is that it is along the path of bliss that we encounter what truly scares us most. This fear is that of meeting our true desires, receiving pleasure, surrendering to it. As opposed to being "too little," we worry that we may be "too much."

So again . . .

Whether you feel you are "too much" or "too little," whether you are by yourself and without the accountability to another person, or whether you are with a partner and risk their judgment, I encourage you to take it slow and be patient with yourself. Be patient with others, too. For once you become more acquainted with the building blocks in each chapter and especially how to bring them together, you will discover that you have built a versatile home that will weather the severest of storms and from which you can keep your bearings while you explore and navigate your wildest dreams and ultimately let go into your highest ecstasies with excitement and success. In that you can trust!

CHAPTER ONE:

BREATH
AND VOICE

YOUR BREATH

Of all the skill sets you can gain, breath is the most basic—yet it is by far the most important. I cannot emphasize this enough. Any yogi, martial artist, athlete, doctor, masseuse, or body specialist worth your time or money will tell you the same thing. You can go without sleep, food, or fluids, or sit improperly or perform a technique incorrectly for a certain amount of time before your body fades out, but never so as quickly as when you go without oxygen to your lungs, blood, or brain. With breath alone, you can stretch, train, strengthen, massage, de-armor, move energy, heal, balance, focus, orgasm, and so much more. Train your breath first, and everything else will follow. Otherwise, everything else will be like the fancy flying kicks in a kung fu movie . . . just for show.

GETTING BACK TO BASICS

Watch a baby breathe. If you do not have one, find a video of one online. Now, really watch how the baby breathes. See, feel, and emulate this and you will have already taken a huge step, potentially the biggest step towards optimizing your sexual performance. Watch how a baby's stomach swells, not just outward like a little Buddha, but watch how the ribs expand to the side. Watch the lower back, as each breath of life is smoothly and calmly cycled through the system before being released as gently as it was accepted. This is the MOST crucial step towards self-discovery that you will take, and the most important skill that you can bring with you from this entire book. BREATHE THE SAME WAY.

This may seem simple at first, but go to the mirror and see for yourself. Watch your face. Then watch the baby's face. Watch your throat and neck. Watch the baby's. Watch your shoulders and chest. Watch the baby's. Watch your stomach, lower back, hands, arms, legs and feet. Think that you are done? You're not. Look into the baby's eyes, the corners of the eyes, and observe the facial expressions. Then note *every* difference there is between yourself and the baby. Good. Can you fully emulate how a baby breathes? Whether your initial response is "yes" or "no," the likely truthful answer is "no." Let's be fully honest here. It has taken the greatest Tai Chi, Qi Gong and yogi masters their lifetime to become proficient in this simple ability. Watch again, and continue learning and implementing.

Babies are expressive, living, breathing, receptive, emotion-filled humans. Be EMOTION-FILLED. By emotion-filled, I'm not saying we should be babies in the sense of crying, screaming, crapping our pants, or making little scenes of drama left and right. No, watch the baby, for unlike the five-year-old who is seeking attention and testing boundaries, an infant expresses their emotions fully, from head to toe, and truly embodies its feelings, inside and out, according to its corporeal needs. As adults, we can fulfill our corporeal needs, but many of us have become largely inexpressive. Our breath is a most basic expression of our state of being. It lets us know the present state of our emotions and health. Watching how someone breathes can gives us insight into another person's state of being. Breath is where we begin our journey to optimize our sex life, and breath will be our tool.

EXERCISE 1: Baby-Belly Breathing

The purpose of this exercise is to bring conscientiousness to your breath until it becomes second nature.

1. Take nine minutes right *now* to sit down and focus on nothing but your breath.

    a. Inhale, feeling your stomach, lower back and ribs swell out in all directions.

    b. Allow your shoulders, neck, head, and hips to gently rock back as the rest of your body remains completely relaxed.

c. Breathe in fully, but allow no tension or strain into your shoulders by forcing air into your lungs. Breathe into your expanding belly.

2. Feel your breath throughout your body: the gentle expansion, the calming release.

3. Feel from the top of your head, down to the tips of your toes, within and without your brain and body—feel the expansive reach and centered release of this universe's most precious gift to you, your unencumbered breath.

EXERCISE 2: **Body Scan**

With this exercise you will practice developing proprioception so that you become accustomed to checking in with and maintaining awareness of the state of your physical body. This is important for avoiding injuries and knowing when to take yourself further.

1. Now take nine minutes to scan your body for any tension, itch, twitch, or need to move.

2. Breathe into the itch or tension. Move, scratch, or adjust as needed, but continue to breathe into any disquietude until the sensation is gone from your body . . . gone from your mind.

3. Take note of any trouble spots that refuse to release, disappear, or that continue to resurface when you repeat the exercise.

    a. We will return to those areas in Exercise 4, as well as in Chapter 3: *Plasticity, Touch, and Technique*, Exercises 25-28.

This is most likely important information, because your body is speaking to you and informing you of where you may have some physical blocks to release.

b. During the body scan, did you notice any change in body temperature? Did you get goose bumps, see colors, or feel pleasure, passion, excitement, comfort, or relaxation? Did you experience the release of tension?

EXERCISE 3: **Emotional Scan**

Here you will practice developing proprioception so that you become accustomed to checking in with and maintaining awareness of your emotions. This is important for establishing your own boundaries, which if violated could lead to unexpected, unintended, and sometimes physically aggressive outbursts or an undermining of your free will when[1] others try to control or impose their will upon you.

1. Repeat Exercise 2 for the same amount of time, except instead of scanning your physical body for tension I invite you to allow yourself to feel your emotional body.

2. Just as before, continue baby-belly breathing, but as you scan your body, allow yourself to become aware of and to feel your emotions. From head to toes, within and without, FEEL.

a. What emotions, stories or thoughts arise as you breathe into and feel your lungs, your heart, your brain, head, face, feet, heels, toes, fingernails, roots of your hairs, genitals, butt, butt hole, penis or vagina?

- Allow yourself to express—with sounds, movements, or words—whatever you feel emotionally.

b. Continue breathing deeper, more profoundly, into the emotion. Feel it, but do not become it or the story it may provide. Instead, like a flowing river, simply let the emotion flow by while you breathe through it, adjusting your position or voice as needed.

c. Take in your emotions and whatever stories may be playing out in your mind, like a fulfilled fisherman with the net still in the water, noting anything that gets caught.

d. Observe and simply return the emotions or stories to the river so they can flow on while you remain constant in your steady breathing for nine minutes or longer.

e. Did any emotions continue to surface? Did they become stronger when you scanned one body part or another? Did you struggle with, or become unable to release the emotions to the river before returning to a state of inner peace? When scanning your body or feeling your emotions, did you find it easy to continue baby-belly breathing? Or did your breath catch at any point or time?

f. Take note, especially noting anywhere in the body you were scanning when one or more of these sensations arose. They will be useful for us, and we can return to them later in the Chapter 3: *Plasticity, Touch, and Technique*, Exercises 21-25, as well as addressing them now in Exercise 4.

EXERCISE 4: **The Gift to Yourself**

In this exercise you will practice developing compassion and non-judgment towards yourself. This way, you become accustomed to nurturing change without beating yourself up, and instead from a position of positivity and reward.

1. For now, simply breathe into whatever you took note of in Exercises 2 and 3, filling your entire body, lungs and stomach for a count of three heartbeats (or three seconds if you cannot yet note your heart beating) and slowly release for nine seconds.

2. Repeat, smiling acknowledgment, love and compassion into whatever tension, emotion or body part you've noted a reaction in until it becomes warm and tingly.

3. Remember to thank your body and mind, as it is simply communicating where and what you may need to address as you prepare yourself for the optimal state of sex.

    a. When you learn to listen to your body, you will understand that it is constantly interacting with your internal and external environment and communicating to you real-time feedback to guide and help you. This line of communication is a gift to yourself.

YOUR VOICE: LET'S HEAR FROM YOU

Now that you have taken the single most important step towards sexual freedom—to breathe fully and unencumbered—this may likely be your most challenging and difficult task . . . giving voice to your sex life.

My 2nd job after finishing my undergraduate degree was working as a social coach. (The first job was as an English teacher.) As a social coach, I was interested in discovering the essential for sparking sexual attraction in interactions. I learned a lot by teaching that year as I traveled around with Wayne Elise,[2] demonstrating and guiding men through the process of meeting a woman at a social gathering, such as at a bar, or as passers-by in life at a grocery store or in a park. One of the many all-too-obvious-yet-greatly-overlooked tips of Wayne's was that we should be more expressive and forthcoming with verbalizing our sentiments and intentions. This can be a challenge and downright scary for many people, who have been taught a political correctness that in some cases can mistake gender-equality for sameness, and gender-respect for neutered interactions. The ability to be sexy and fun, while making others feel the same about themselves, celebrates our gender differences by exciting and further increasing the polarity of the magnetic pull between these differences. Wayne is an artist in his ability to inspire charisma, and teach others how to most enjoyably converse and incite sexual excitement by expressing their sexual intentions in a way that is fun and sexy for the person listening. It is interesting to consider how this applies when we move beyond words and our acts become distinctly physical.

I have practiced with, witnessed, de-armored, massaged and attended seminars and workshops with some of the most sexually experienced, elite, knowledgeable and wonderfully juicy tantrikas, dakinis, dakas and gurus around the world. Yet, if I were to note the most overlooked factor missing from practice and activity (my own included) then it would be that of voice . . . the practice of genuinely voicing one's arousal and full-fledged sexuality. I can't tell you how many times my wife has reminded me in the throes of sexual passion and enjoyment "breathe and let me hear you." I can also tell you how much this statement, when my mind and body are not open, challenges my ego. Oftentimes, when I'm closed, my initial unspoken reaction is something to the effect of, "Please shut up and let me be how I am." Let's examine this statement for a moment.

How we normally are as humans, when comfortable and feeling open, is in general communicative creatures who allow themselves to be heard. It is typically the socially shunned and awkward who struggle or refuse to voice their feelings, thoughts and desires. Most of us in any social gathering, except a funeral, chat our butts off, maybe even ad nauseum, to our listeners and our own exhaustion. So why the stark difference when it comes to sex, in what should be the most social, intimate and interactive act humans perform? Well the answer lies in the former part of the response: "shut up."

Start now by taking full baby-belly breaths and allow yourself to shift in your seat and realize that a response of "shut up" to this imagined or real moment of sexual honesty from your partner is how you or I are . . . "shut up" and needing to be opened. For those of you who are socially awkward and struggle to communicate, you may actually find voicing in the bedroom to be extremely liberating, as it doesn't have to involve words and is often most effective when it does not.

MAKING NOISE VS. BEING EXPRESSIVE

Now many here will likely have a secondary reaction such as, "Okay, so what voice or sounds should I make?" I'm not telling you to fake some banshee-like, high-pitched shrilling sound you last saw on a free porn website, nor is it the point for your neighbors to hear you. Though, I might just point out that your neighbor already hears you yelling over your mobile phone, as well the gory violence from the action film you play at high volume. In fact, the sound of you genuinely enjoying the act of love might be a pleasant change.

The point is for us to express ourselves to our playmate and to liberate our repressed "shut up" self. Are you still struggling with the thought of this challenge? No worries. Almost everyone has found this difficult at first and from time to time. The good news is that with the practice of a few exercises this becomes quite natural and extremely liberating. Take some baby-belly breaths and continue reading. Exercise 5 is geared specifically to help you with this.

On the opposite end of the Social-Spectrum from "The Awkwardly Silent" is the "Chatty Kathy or Charlie" who just speaks to speak and is otherwise plagued with what one of my friends from high school termed "verbal diarrhea." Whereas the expressive and *open* person and the expressive yet *closed* person are true opposites, the character plagued with verbal diarrhea and the silently awkward person are two sides of the same inexpressive coin. Both are awkward, and both create "noise." *Noise* in the sense I mean here is "white noise." It is unfocused, distracting, non-expressive communication that impedes and inhibits interaction. As such, you should not make "white noise" or become the "Chatty Charlie or Kathy" of the bedroom, just for the attention or benefit of sugarcoating your partner's ego. Remember the purpose of voicing is to truly and genuinely express yourself with sound, to *open up* yourself and your partner. In Chinese reflexology there is a direct connection between the throat and vagina/penis. When your vocal chords vibrate, the throat and the genitals begin to release tension and open up to greater sensation and higher levels of pleasure. When you become comfortable voicing your pleasure and can likewise encourage your partner's comfort in voicing theirs, you will have already placed yourself in the category of "superior lover." Let us now venture into discovering, through exploration, what is optimal.

SING FOR ME

I never really was one of those kids who thought girls had cooties. I have always been, as far back as I can remember, sexual. If I had to be labeled, it would most likely be some form of philogynist. Where most boys want to tease or even hit girls, I was curious about kissing them and about what pleasure I might find with them. As a teenager, when most guys dreamed or bragged of getting blowjobs, I read books on massage, female orgasms, and how to achieve multiple male orgasms. In military high school, college, and still to this day with the many males I meet in their 40s and 50s, I find men who fantasize about sleeping with [*insert celebrity crush*] or having a threesome with [*aforementioned celebrity*] + [*some other celebrity*].

I soon noted that my fantasies were somewhat different and rarely left to mere imagination. My dream and fantasy of ultimately spending a lifetime with a woman, exploring with her everything the world had to offer, oriented me, even at an early age, to be around girls in such a way that made me a favorite with parents.

At other times, my sexual curiosity and imagination made me less of a favorite, as was the case when I was only five years old. My slightly-older next-door neighbor and I decided to play a fantasy game that we had come up with in the spur of the moment with the toys we had present. Making use of my new, shiny set of handcuffs, her backyard fence, and our genital curiosity, the game was some sort of mix between "doctor" and "cops and robbers." As we took turns being handcuffed and exploring "the captive's" sex, I was captivated by how much her vagina looked like a deep-red, blushing flower. I was even more impressed by the intense heat her flower transmitted to my finger (the heat felt like it was going into the core of my finger and not just on to my skin's surface), and I recall how much we both found this exploration so intriguing.

Her parents, however, did not.

When she gleefully recounted the experience to them, they forbade her to play or speak with me. Years later, well after I had returned from living in Portugal with my parents and brother, she and I attended the same junior high school. We had a good laugh about it. Around the same time as the hand-cuffing exploration, my parents were less than thrilled when they walked into their bedroom and found me conducting what can best be described as a mixed gender *sexploration* workshop with my friends.

I never felt ashamed by these adventures, though I didn't like embarrassing my parents.

I did, however, puzzle over why the adults were so upset, and how guilt seemed to consume my friends afterwards. Looking back, I have come to believe that often our own sexual inhibitions and stifled fantasies are by-products of the reactive judgments from our parents' own discomfort, as well as the epoch's surrounding social stigmas when it comes to the topic of sex. If it is difficult to even speak of sex in a person's family, then it is no wonder that voicing one's sexual stimulation can be such a challenge. Be it for fear of judgment or self-reinforced shame, the voice in your head may be outshouting the voice of your sexual body.

One of the fantasies I had in my early 20s, when I first started to have sex, was to be ridden by a singer with an oper-atic voice while she sung full blast. I lived out this fantasy some years later while finishing my Master's degree. The woman who fulfilled that fantasy was a professional blues singer from whom I was renting a room. After taking some moments and two attempts to find her voice with me inside her . . . and then a few more to coordinate it with her movement, we had great fun. I believe this must have left a lasting impression on me, as years later my wife and I had an epiphany that became a turning point in our sex life.

My wife and I, after much wonderful practice with many of the same exercises and realizations you will hopefully gain in this book, were passionately involved in sex. We were very connected and experiencing profound pleasure. Her face was relaxed. Her cheeks were flushed. As her jaw went limp and her lips parted, her mouth opened. Without thinking, the words spilled from me, "Your body is an instrument! Sing for me!" Far different from the singer's melodic, composed vocals, my wife's entire being erupted with erotic liberation. The most natural, uniquely precious moans, sighs, heavy breaths and expressions of pure ecstasy began to emanate from this magnificent woman as she began transforming before my eyes. Waves of orgasmic pleasure began to cascade out from my Empress's throat and chest, to enrapture her from her head to sprawled toes like an embodied instrument proliferating note after majestic note in an improvisational concert of the finest quality. My body in turn began to resonate and quake in harmonious bliss. From here forward, the incorporation of voice, combined with breath, became a cornerstone in the development of our sexual practice.

YOUR INSTRUMENT

Our mind, unlike a driver disconnected from the outside world and cocooned within an automobile, is not merely a brain interpreting and computing the abstract words of other drivers through its rear-view mirror, but instead is a fully embodied instrument that interacts directly in concert with the resonant expressions of those within its surrounding field. This should be rather obvious: one person can say something, and the cadence, resonance and delivery in his or her voice can stress you, while another person can say the exact same thing and their words can melt you like butter over fresh-baked bread. We are not an isolated brain interpreting fixed signs at a disconnected distance and performing programmed, computer-like functions. We are much more. We are musical instruments resonating in accord with the universe. Voice, verbal or non-verbal, creates the notes that pluck at our soul and opens our hearts.

Hopefully, you are at least curious to address the next logical question. "How do I activate my voice?" Like any instrument, let's start by learning its notes. If ever you ask one of the many people I have helped *open up,* they will likely recall the following basic exercises. I hope they serve you well as you discover the vast potential of empowering your sex life with these basic, yet foundational, tools of your breath and voice.

EXERCISE 5: **Resonant Voicing**

The body, like an instrument, resonates with different tones in different places. A simple YouTube search for chakra tones will even give you the hertz corresponding to each of your body's basic seven chakras.

1. Begin by taking in a full baby-belly breath, gently lifting your chin so you fill your lungs to maximum capacity.

2. As you release your breath, voice each tone until your breath is fully expired, starting with your root chakra and working your way up and back down each chakra, one by one.

   a. You will naturally expel the air fastest at the beginning of the exhalation, so be sure to focus from the very first molecular release of air for a slow, steady and smooth release.

3. Repeat the sound for each chakra seven times. Focus on creating as much vibration as possible with your vocal chords and feeling for resonance in the corresponding chakra.

4. Note all body or emotional sensations as you did with Exercises 1-4.

5. Experiment with volume, explosiveness, continuity, and rate. Note the different effects they have.

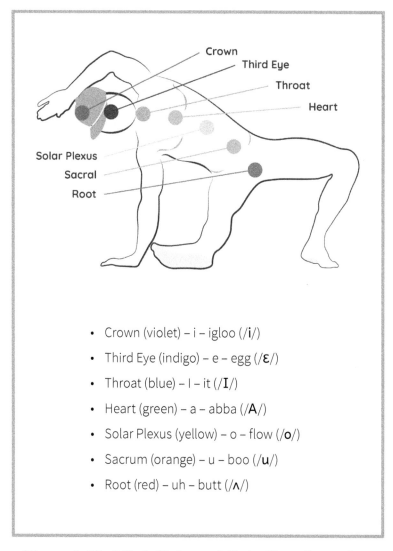

- Crown (violet) – i – igloo (/i/)
- Third Eye (indigo) – e – egg (/ɛ/)
- Throat (blue) – I – it (/I/)
- Heart (green) – a – abba (/A/)
- Solar Plexus (yellow) – o – flow (/o/)
- Sacrum (orange) – u – boo (/u/)
- Root (red) – uh – butt (/ʌ/)

Diagram 1: The 7 Basic Chakras and Chakra Tones. Do not close your mouth to make the /u/ sound of the "w." It is a pure /o/.

ADDITIONAL TIPS FOR IDENTIFYING RESONANCE

These are your palms' kidney points where your chi enters and exits your hands. We will return to it in Chapter 4: *Power and Stamina*, when working with your power. You will use these points to heighten awareness and proprioception in your hands for interacting with yourself as well as others.

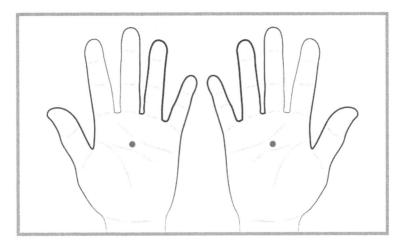

Diagram 2: Open Palms with Lao Gung Points

EXERCISE 6: **Additional Tip #1 (solo practice)**

1. Center your Lao Gung point from either hand on your root chakra.
2. Proceed according to steps 2, 3, and 4 from Exercise 5, following your voice's progression along the chakra scale with your hand.
   a. Feel for a concentrated vibration in your palm.

3. In one breath and voice, alternate between your root and crown chakras as they provide the largest contrast between each other. This will allow you to most easily identify the difference in where the resonant vibration is concentrated.

4. In one breath and continuous voice, try to voice the entire chakra scale from root to crown.

5. Now see if you can voice the entire scale from bottom to top and back down again.

   a. While keeping your hand centered over the chakra, note if you can continue to feel the vibration in your hand as you bring it further away from your body.

EXERCISE 7: **Additional Tip #2 (partner practice)**

1. With a partner, repeat Exercise 6, except place your Lao Gung point on their corresponding chakras, as they voice them.

2. As they exhale and project energy out through their voice, you should inhale and feel for the concentrated vibration coming from their chakra into your palm (i.e. If they voice their heart chakra, then your Lao Gung point should be over their heart chakra).

3. Now, you exhale, projecting energy back into them from your Lao Gung point while voicing the corresponding chakra. They should inhale and absorb your energy.

4. Repeat nine times and then switch roles.

CHAPTER TWO:

POSTURE AND MOVEMENT

YOUR POSTURE

I was a sophomore at the University of Michigan. After a successful freshman year boxing for the university, I had qualified for nationals. I had been boxing for only one season yet had TKO'ed (Technical Knockout) the former regional champion in the second round of the USA regional championships. I went the distance in the championship fight against Navy's up and coming best, who eventually ended up getting second or third in the nation. However, when the final bell rang and the match was over I did not receive the ring judges' decisions after what could be termed as nothing other than an all-out slugfest. NAVY's team captain came to my locker and personally congratulated me on the fight, for as he put it, their boxer had a reputation for KO's (knockouts) and removing heads. This was something I had personally borne witness to in his previous regional fights. As second in my region, I had qualified for nationals and was automatically placed in the nation's top eight intercollegiate boxers for my weight class.

I had joined the team, however, to learn how to fight beyond my wrestling background, throw a punch and see how I parried or handled being hit. This I accomplished to my satisfaction, so I decided I would focus on finals and chose to use my head and hands for other purposes.

I didn't have as much as a bruise or bloodied nose after an entire season, so you can imagine my coach's surprise when I decided not to go to Vegas to compete for the national title. Considering he was losing his star rookie, he handled my decision well. I had met my goals and knew I could handle myself on the streets. On a deeper level I wanted to now delve into more internal martial arts and harness something of which I only had begun to hear about: chi. After visiting several sports clubs, none of which really seemed to offer much practical application, I came across Pencak Silat. Sitting on the side of a room in a small tantric Buddhist temple, I witnessed my first Silat class. I was intrigued by the fifty-year-old guru who led the group. The class sweated, strained, and shook from head to toe as they worked through what looked like simple movements, albeit moves low to the ground. The guru, however, moved with ease, agility, grace, and precision while delivering multiple lightning-speed blows. Rather effortlessly, he struck at will with power and at angles that confounded the mind, all the while floating like a slow-motion butterfly with a smile across his face.

I sat and waited to join. Eventually he approached me as the class continued to practice the series of steps he had just shown them. What he said next has stuck with me to this day: "One must first learn to breath. With proper breath one can obtain proper posture. With proper posture one can maintain balance. Only in balance can one move freely. Then and only then, with proper breath, posture, balance, and freedom of movement, can one generate true speed and power."

You can apply this back-to-basics method to every physical discipline and quite easily extend it to all aspects of your life. Even meditation, the maintenance of any state, or the shift from one state to a more centered one (which some consider a primarily mental discipline), depends on these factors. It is also the reason why I have structured this book as I have. In the previous chapter you were introduced to breath and voice; now let me introduce you to bedroom postures.

SEXUAL POSTURING

Postures:
1. Horse Stance
2. Horse on Knees
3. Horse on Hands and Knees
4. Horse on Side
5. Horse on Back

POSTURE #1: HORSE STANCE

The Horse Stance is probably the most basic, foundational, yet incorrectly enacted posture in all martial arts. It is seemingly simple, yet like baby-belly breathing it can take years to truly master. Fortunately, precise instruction will suffice to help your body most naturally cycle energy in bed. Postures #2-5 are variations of the Horse Stance. Though the body's orientation is changed, its relative alignment is basically the same. If you have trouble with this posture at first, you can get a feel for it by practicing the steps with your back flat against the wall.

EXERCISE 8: Horse Stance

1. Stand with your feet together. With open hands and thumbs forward, allow your arms to hang directly down from your shoulders, perpendicular to the floor.

2. Line up the outside of your feet with your fingers, and ensure the outer sides of your feet are completely parallel to each other. For many, this may feel quite awkward at first. You may even think you are standing pigeon-toed. However, this is actually because most of us are used to walking and standing slightly penguin-toed (toes turned out), which is also why so many of us have lower back and hip pain.

3. Rock onto your heels and turn your toes out so the center points of the balls of your feet are at a forty-five degree angle from the center of your heels.

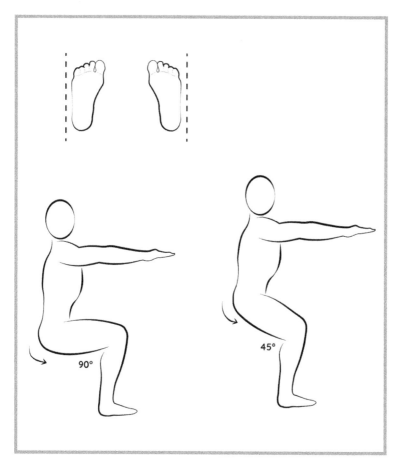

Diagram 3: Feet Posture in Horse Stance. The outside of the feet are parallel. The feet are more than shoulder-width apart.

4. Return balance to the center point of the balls of your feet once again, and align the outsides of your feet so they are parallel.

5. Without moving your feet, squat straight down. Your feet will probably want to turn out and shift your weight to your heels . . . don't. Maintain your balance over the balls of your feet and keep the outsides parallel to one another.

6. Notice the alignment of your spine. From the crown of your head, through your spine, and down to your sacrum, your back should be flat and fully perpendicular to the floor. It will feel like you are tucking in your butt, but only do so until your sacrum is perpendicular to the floor.

7. Look straight ahead with your knees bent at a forty-five to ninety-degree angle, depending on your ability. Glance down with only your eyes. Your knees should be positioned so you can see all your toes except your big toes.

8. For the purpose of this drill, extend your arms with palms facing out so they are parallel to the floor.

9. Practice holding this stance for three, six or nine minutes, belly breathing throughout this exercise.

   a. Beginners in martial arts will gradually work their way up to sixty minutes and several minutes beyond that in the morning and again at night to truly internalize the stance.

   b. To get a feel of this posture and exercise, you can repeat steps 1-8 with your entire back flat against the wall.

EXERCISE 9: **Additional Tip for Lower Back Pain Relief**

I would be doing you a disservice if while practicing Horse Stance I did not make you aware of how it can really help you correct your posture, and especially relieve pain from your lower back and hips.

1. As opposed to using your squatting muscles (quadriceps) by fighting directly against gravity like most of us gym rats do, your feet should feel rooted into the ground. Bow your legs out.

2. Have someone push in on the outer sides of your knees. While maintaining proper posture, resist collapsing your knees in that your big toe remains covered by your knee as detailed in the last sentence of Exercise 8, *Horse Stance*.

3. When resisting, do not push out with your knees. Instead, push from your sacrum and hips using your butt muscles. Feel your lower back open as your thighs rotate in towards your groin.

4. If you can, then sink deeper into the stance while your friend is still providing resistance. This can be most relieving to those of us who suffer from lower back and hip pain.

POSTURE #2 HORSE ON KNEES

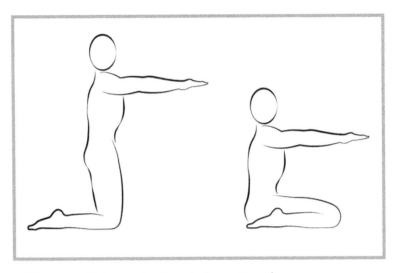

Diagram 4 (alternative 1 and alternative 2):
Performing Horse on Knees

EXERCISE 10: **Horse on Knees**

1. From Posture #1, allow your knees to follow a natural arc forward until they reach the floor, ground, mat, or bed.

  a. Take care not to hurt your knees.

2. Baby-breathe for three minutes, practicing your chakra tones. Note that your back and spine should still be relatively flat and perpendicular to the surface on which you are situated.

POSTURE #3 HORSE ON HANDS AND KNEES

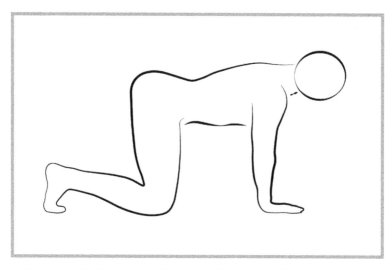

Diagram 5: Performing Horse on Hands and Knees

EXERCISE 11: **Horse on Hand and Knees**

1. From Posture #2, extend your arms straight forward with your palms facing out. Bend forward at your hips, and be sure to catch yourself with your hands before you face plant.

2. With your arms and thighs perpendicular to the floor, and your neck and back parallel to the floor, begin belly breathing and chakra sounding. Really focus on using gravity in this position to fully relax and expand your belly towards the earth. With each inhalation, feel your belly expand to its full extent.

POSTURE #4 HORSE ON SIDE

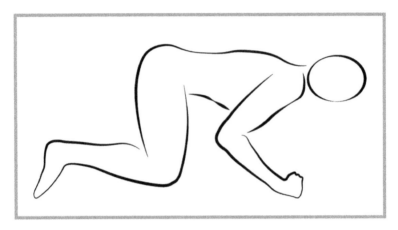

Diagram 6: Horse on Side (bird's-eye view)

EXERCISE 12: Horse on Side

1. From Posture #3, place your left shoulder where your left hand was, and extend your left arm to your right side, across your chest, and just behind your right hand.

    a. Keeping your right palm flat on the ground, your right arm will naturally bend at the elbow to approximately a ninety-degree angle.

2. Rotate further so you place your left hip where your left knee is.

3. Allow your right leg to rotate up as you sweep your left leg across your underside and towards the right. Finish by rotating onto your side.

    a. Maintain the ninety-degree bend at the knees and the flat back from Posture #3.

4. Belly breathe and sound your chakras.

5. Place your right palm where it was before and rotate your chest back towards the floor.

6. Supporting yourself with your right hand and arm strength, lift your chest enough so that you can place your left palm where your left shoulder was located on the floor.

7. Pushing yourself up, rotate your hips back again to the left so that you return to Posture #3: Horse on Hands and Knees.

POSTURE #5 HORSE ON BACK

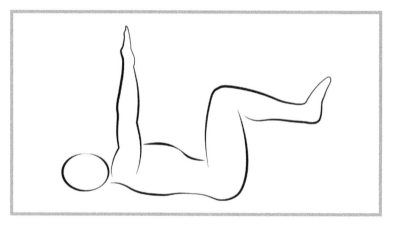

Diagram 7: Performing Horse on Back

EXERCISE 13: **Horse on Back**

1. Assume Posture #4, Horse on Side, and note which hip and shoulder is toward the ceiling.

2. From Posture #4, rotate simultaneously the hip and shoulder which are toward the ceiling so that you end up with your back flat on the floor.

3. With your feet off the ground, maintain the ninety-degree bend at your knees so your shins are parallel to the floor.

4. With arms and palms extended up and out towards the ceiling or sky, practice baby-belly breathing and resonant voicing.

    a. Ensure with each breath that your lungs, belly, back and genitals are breathed into and expanded to their maximum capacity.

EXERCISE 14: **Connecting the Postures**

Once you have become comfortable with belly-breathing and voicing in each of the postures, the following simple exercise can be a fun practice that will help develop a sense of connection and fluidity between each posture.

1. Begin in Posture #1, Horse Stance, and start breathing into and voicing your root chakra.

2. With each exhale, voice your root chakra and shift postures in ascending order (i.e. #1, #2, #3, both sides of Posture #4, and then #5).

3. When you reach the place in Posture #5 where you're on your back, lean your head towards your left shoulder.

    a. This will bring your left ear closer to your left shoulder and create a separation between your right ear and your right shoulder.

4. In the separation between your right ear and your right shoulder, perform a reverse somersault by rolling your knees straight back over your shoulders towards the ground behind your head.

5. Land back on your hands and knees in Posture #3, Horse on Hands and Knees.

6. Come up to Posture #2, Horse on Knees, and then finish by standing up into Posture #1, Horse Stance.

7. Repeat steps 1-5 until you can move fluidly between all the postures.

   a. Note that each time you perform the somersault in step 5, you will be facing a different direction.

8. If you are cycling through the postures and wish to finish in the same direction, then before performing the somersault in step 4, simply rotate your body 180 degrees by spinning on your flat back so your head ends up where your feet were.

YOUR MOVEMENT: THE DANCE WITHIN (AKA THE MOTION IN YOUR OCEAN)

Ever since I was a kid, I have, on more than several occasions, felt energy throughout my body that caused my spine to undulate like ripples over still water. I never knew there was a word for what I was experiencing. I simply thought this was something everyone experienced. I first heard the term "kundalini" from a Danish classmate at Aarhus University. She had been at a meditation retreat in England where her kundalini had opened for her. Nevertheless, my own formal introduction to kundalini energy and how to free it in others came several years later when my wife signed us up for an introductory tantra workshop. There, two experienced bodyworkers gave me a hard touch, external de-armoring to open my kundalini. I stripped down to my boxer briefs and noted how good it felt as I removed my three-piece suit, tie and dress shoes. The session was even more phenomenal, leaving me filled with laughter and energy surging throughout my body.

Curious to learn more about kundalini, my wife and I attended a Saturday evening workshop in the small town of Egtved, just outside of Kolding, Denmark. It was led by a gifted physiotherapist by the name of Henrik Frydendahl. For a few hundred Danish kroner, he was basically giving away the course by charging just enough to cover his expenses for drinks and snacks. After introducing the group to some theory, he broke us participants into groups of four. Under his expert guidance three people would be led through how to apply various trigger point and tapping techniques while the fourth person lay before them, receptive. We rotated until everyone had had a chance to receive. It provoked tremendous emotional releases, and left attendees feeling free in their minds and bodies. Some people were catharticaly crying, having let go of years of stress as the group cuddled them. Others were left pleasurably writhing as if their spines had become enlivened tracks of undulating pleasure. Henrik noticed my ability to work on others. After the course ended, he asked if I wanted to assist him with further workshops. It was the birth of a lasting friendship, and I gained much experience opening, playing with, and discovering what was possible with this life force called "kundalini."

One woman had struggled to overcome her daily addiction to drinking several liters of sugary sodas since being a teenager. After only one session, she went several weeks without even a craving for the beverage. It was a first for her. Another woman regained her sex drive, much to her boyfriend's satisfaction. He was a bodybuilder, built like Adonis, but felt impotent in himself and his ability to arouse his partner. Eager to experience and learn about kundalini energy, he signed up the very next day for the following workshop.

On and on I witnessed, or was told of by participants, numerous success stories where people overcame personal psychosomatic challenges. Unfortunately, for would-be attendees, around six months later Henrik received a job offer too good to turn down. The work would not allow him the time needed to continue our partnership for these weekend workshops. Nevertheless, all the work with my own kundalini and that of others brought about a realization. It was this sensation, dancing through my spine, which had brought me to seek out ways to harness my chi and work with my breath. Kundalini inspired my love of improvisational dance and music. It maintained my actively, exploratory perspective on sex as an art, and it is likely the reason why I was never really satisfied by the status quo's complacency to simply scratch a sexual itch when it arose.

This energy has existed under many names and there are just as many methods for how to awaken, tap into, and strengthen one's kundalini. Some ways are forceful, others gentler. As a rule of thumb, you should avoid those hard touch forms which leave heavy bruising, especially along the body's centerline, running down the back and front side of your body between your crown and root chakras. Bruises are a sign of damaged tissue and often result in blocking energy as opposed to releasing it. Breath, posture, and the following exercises are often enough to put us in touch with this incredible life force that is already trickling, or even continually streaming, through us. By taking the time and insisting on a steadfast effort to train, learn, play with, and ultimately wield this energy, we can begin to revolutionize our perspective on, and experience of, sex. Once blockage and debris are cleared away, be it physical or psychological scarring—and one normally begets the other—our trickling streams will transform into ocean tides that surge and dance.

WARMING UP THE SPINE

Let's begin with a few simple exercises to warm up the spine. The key to every one of these preparatory exercises is to move slowly at first. In cadence with your breath, connect to and identify each vertebra, joint and muscle used until they are all warm and tingly. These exercises can be found in various practices such as Yoga, Tai Chi, Qi Gong, Tantra, and Dance. Each practice has its own slight variations, depending on whether your intention and embodied art is martial, healing, or simply aesthetic. The purposes here are for improving one's sexual pleasure and, ultimately, for the wealth of your health and prosperity.

WARM UP #1: THE SPAGHETTI TWIST

This exercise will help prevent any injuries that may arise when rotating your shoulders, wrists, or along the spine.

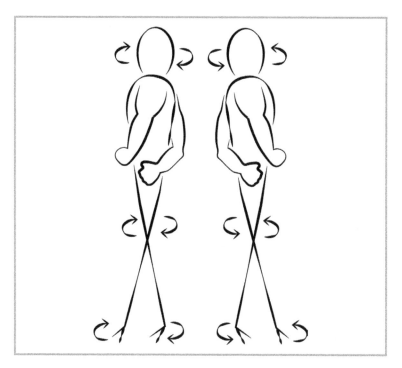

Diagram 8: Performing the Spaghetti Twist

EXERCISE 15: **The Spaghetti Twist**

1. Align your feet, as in step 2 of Exercise #8, *Horse Stance*.

2. Twisting from the force in your hips, wring your spine like a towel, keeping it straight and erect while the rest of your body remains limp.

3. With each twist of your hips, look back 180 degrees as you turn back and forth from one side to the other.

4. Allow your hips and feet to twist as well.

   a. Ensure that your feet pivot on the balls of your feet, not the heels.

5. Your arms should hang limp like spaghetti, moving only from the centrifugal force of your twisting hips and spine.

   a. As you twist left, your arms should naturally swing left. As you complete the twist, your left arm will swing back and slap your lower back with the back of your left palm. Your right arm naturally swings around your front side, slapping your left side with the open palm of your right hand. The opposite should occur as you twist right.

6. Your exhalation should reach completion as your twist finishes; your hands will slap to a stop, and you will be looking back 180 degrees.

7. Inhale as you begin twisting in the other direction. You should reach full lung capacity when you are looking straight forward. Your exhalation begins as you twist in the other direction.

   a. This is to be executed in a relaxed, fluid motion.

8. Repeat nine times in each direction or until your spine feels warm and tingly.

WARM-UP #2: THE BRIDGE

This exercise will help prevent any injuries that may arise when bending over or standing up erect.

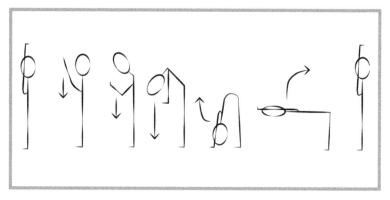

Diagram 9: Performing the Bridge

EXERCISE 16: **The Bridge**

1. Align your feet as in step 2 of Exercise 8, *Horse Stance.*

2. Inhale, lifting your arms so they are fully extended up. With your palms open and facing out, complete your intake of breath.

3. As you exhale, allow your hands to slowly lower down, not out and down, but straight down, as if by gravity and directly in front of your face. Slowly follow your body's profile.

4. As your palms pass at eye level, your head should follow by curling forward and in, one vertebra at a time. Starting from the top vertebra and proceeding all the way down to the bottom of your spine, time the curling of your vertebrae with the passing of your hands.

5. Your exhale should reach its completion as your palms touch the ground, or when you can go no further.

6. When fully extended down, your neck should be hanging relaxed with your arms and shoulders resting loosely by your ears as you gaze toward your legs.

7. As you begin to inhale, use the muscles in the middle of your back to lift your extended arms until your upper body is parallel to the ground.

8. Your body should be bent at a ninety-degree angle from your waist, with your arms fully extended out and palms facing out.

9. Using only the lower muscles of your back, lift yourself like a bridge from the waist up while keeping everything fully extended. Finish your inhalation when your body is fully erect and has reached the position detailed in step 2.

10. Repeat nine times.

WARM-UP #3: FETCH THE WATER

This exercise will help prevent any injuries that may arise when bending over or standing up erect with a rotated spine.

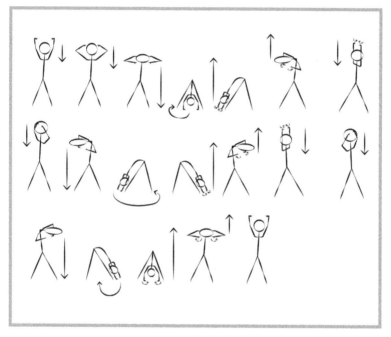

Diagram 10: Performing Fetch the Water

EXERCISE 17: **Fetch the Water**

1. Align your feet as in step 2 of Exercise 8, *Horse Stance.*

2. Inhale, lifting your arms so they are fully extended up.

    a. To correctly position your hands, open your palms. Face them in towards each other, then bend them from your wrists towards one another. Your fingers should be pointing to each other with your palms facing down and parallel to the ground.

3. As you exhale, allow your hands to slowly lower straight down. As in the previous exercise, do so once again as if by gravity, directly in front of your face, and following your body's profile.

4. When your palms, which are still facing down, pass eye level, your head should follow by curling forward and in, one vertebra at a time. Starting from the top vertebra and proceeding all the way down to the bottom, time the curling of your vertebrae with the passing of your hands.

5. Your exhalation should reach its completion as your palms touch the ground or you can go no further.

6. When fully extended down, your neck should be hanging down, relaxed, with your arms and shoulders resting closely by your ears as you gaze toward your legs with your palms turned out towards the ground.

7. Twist from your waist to your left without moving your feet until your hands are parallel with and next to the outside of your left foot.

8. Turn both of your palms up and with your inhalation begin to raise your hands up the outside of your left leg.

9. Once your hands reach your lowest vertebra, start to uncurl your back one vertebra at a time while still remaining twisted towards your left leg.

10. Time the uncurling of your vertebra with the passing of your hands, then inhale.

11. With the completion of your inhalation, turn your palms up and away with the fingers of your hands still pointing towards one another.

12. Turn your palms down and remain facing left. Repeat steps 3-11 along the left side of your body nine times (without twisting at step 7 since you are already facing left).

13. After the ninth time, repeat steps 3-7, except from your left side twist over to your right side.

14. Repeat the exercise nine times before returning to the center and coming up.

WARM-UP #4: THE CLOCK

This is an exercise with which most dancers will be familiar. It teaches you how to isolate and move your hips, each step becoming progressively more difficult. Start slowly and gradually build up your speed for fun. More importantly, this exercise will serve as a reference point for the position of your hips and how to move in later exercises.

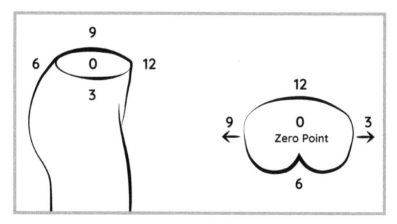

Diagram 11: The Movements of The Clock

EXERCISE 18: **The Clock**

1. Just to orient yourself, place your feet about 10-12 centimeters (3-4 inches) away from the wall. Place your upper and lower back flat against the wall so there is no space between the wall and your lower and upper back. Note where your hips are, as we will refer to this position as *neutral* or being at the *zero point*. Rocking yours hips up and forward we will call this the twelve o'clock position. Rocking backwards, so your lower back comes off the wall, we will call this the six o'clock position, with three o'clock to the right and nine o'clock to the left.

2. Now step away from the wall, and with your feet shoulder-width apart, bring your hips to the zero point. Notice how your spine is in the same position described in step 6 of Exercise 8, *Horse Stance.*

3. Practice rocking your hips forwards and backwards from your twelve o'clock to your six o'clock position, using your lower back and butt muscles. Do so nine times or until you are comfortable with the motion.

4. Practice rocking your hips side to side from your three o'clock to your nine o'clock position. Do so nine times or until you are comfortable with the motion.

5. Now practice rocking your hips forward to your twelve o'clock and return to the zero point, then rock right to the three o'clock and return to the zero point, then six, nine, and again twelve o'clock, always returning to the zero point between each position on the clock. Do nine full rounds before going in the opposite direction (counterclockwise) from twelve to nine, six, and three before returning to twelve.

6. Repeat step 5, except this time do not return to the zero point in between the different points. Do so nine times in both directions.

7. Lastly repeat step 6, except this time smooth out the movement between the points so that your hips make isolated clockwise circles. Do so 21 times and then another 21 times counter clockwise.

    a. By isolated circles, it is meant that you should not bend at the *waist*. In addition, your shoulders and knees should remain relatively stable so that they are not moving back and forth.

THE KUNDALINI DANCE

The key to the Kundalini Dance is to find freedom in movement so every micro movement becomes more micronized and effortless. Meanwhile, the undulating effect in your spine is one of an ever-increasing inertial energy that amplifies until you no longer know if it is you, the dance, the music, or the energy you have tapped into that is causing you to move.

EXERCISE 19: Seated Kundalini Activation

The purpose of this exercise is to begin in a relaxed and seated position so as to most easily get a feeling for the motion. Sit up straight at the edge of your seat so only your butt is on the chair. Plant your feet on the floor shoulder-width apart.

1. Breathe in as you rock your hips into the six o'clock position.

2. Like a ripple, as you rock your hips backwards, allow the curve in your lower back to travel up your spine and into the base of your skull, until your stomach, then chest come forward, followed by the rocking back of your shoulders, neck, then head.

3. Again, like a ripple, as you rock your hips forwards allow the rounding out of your lower back to travel up your spine and into the base of your skull, as your stomach, then chest, curl in, followed by the rocking forward of your shoulders, neck, then head.

4. The overall effect on your spine should be a wave or undulating, snake-like motion. Feel the heat generated by the movement and belly breathing.

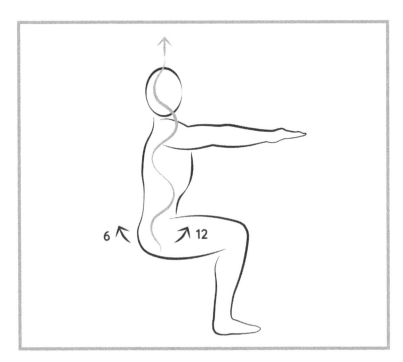

Diagram 12: Performing the Seated Kundalini Dance

EXERCISE 20: **Improvisational Kundalini Dancing**

~~~~~~

The movement of Kundalini Dancing is the same as that in the Seated Kundalini Activation except that it is performed in each of the sexual postures. For the purposes of this exercise, begin in Posture #3, Horse on Hands and Knees. It will naturally free your hips and spine to undulate as well as allow your belly, chest and breath to expand to maximum capacity. Later, when you are familiar with the motion and can easily access your sexual energy, this exercise can be practiced in any position, whether static with feet planted, or walking around your living room. You may even surprise yourself in public, when your kundalini subtly starts to tingle for no apparent reason at all or in response to a chance sexual arousal.

1. Prepare an environment and/or mindset wrought with eroticism.
2. Make a favorite music playlist with sexy beats. The first song should be soft and slow with each following song's beat building up in intensity and metric rate.
3. Press *play.*
4. Begin by focusing on your breathing and try timing it to the beat.
5. Allow your voice to project freely as you exhale, and once again time it to the beat. If no particular sound seems natural, then rhythmically sound out your root chakra to the beat of the music.
6. Incorporate the movement with your breath and sound. Allow the movement to take over as your thoughts turn off, submitting to the sensations, pleasures and eroticism coursing through your body and vibrating in your voice.

7. As your kundalini dances, allow your body to begin rotating through the sexual postures as described in Exercise 14, *Connecting the Postures*.

8. Allow yourself to explore and to become the movements as if in the act of sex.

9. Once you have become familiar with the movements and can easily rotate through the postures, take note how you feel in your physical, as well as your emotional body, just as you did in the first Exercises 1-4.

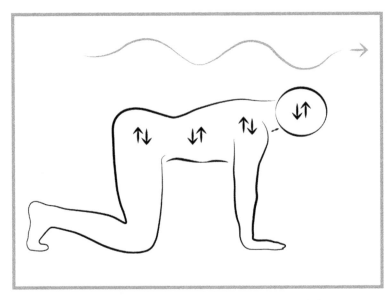

Diagram 13: The Movements of the Dancing Kundalini

CHAPTER THREE:

PLASTICITY, TOUCH, AND TECHNIQUE

YOUR TOUCH: HEALING HANDS

The cognitive sciences have been making progressive leaps and bounds forward in the fields of psychology, neuroscience, neurochemistry, linguistics, language acquisition, emotions, musicology, and philosophy (to name just a few advancements). By in large, much of this is due to the paradigm shift and breaking away from the false dichotomy of mind vs. body, and into the more accurate and holistic understanding of embodiment. *Embodiment* refers to the concept that the mind *is* the body. This means that the mind is not confined to one region of the body, such as the brain. Instead, the entire body is mindful in that our body, not just the brain, enables our sense-making and direct interaction with the world. In fact, even the concept of *an embodied mind* is quickly becoming archaic as the term gives way to the more accurate one of *extended mind*. The extended mind not only dispels the false dichotomy of mind vs. body but builds upon the concept of the embodied mind. The extended mind moves us beyond the egocentric perspective that "the mind is an island" and into the greater truth that our minds are inter-linked. Science acknowledges both the autonomy of our mind's embodiment, yet also concedes that the mind is part of a collec-tively mindful pulse that manifests as our culture, and shapes our personalities and perspectives.

In the same vein, Max Wertheimer's philosophical contri-bution of *gestalt* is finally emerging as prevalent throughout the sciences, with the simple truth that the whole is more than the sum of its parts. Even the "Western" medical community, with its take on health and the body, is opening itself to the more holistic approach of "Eastern" medical study, as well as the likes of Thomas Myers and his well-documented research into the myofascial system, giving a gestalt approach to physiother-apy, as explained in his book *Anatomy Trains*. The dissected per-spective of anatomy has been replaced. Myers and others are solving chronic pains, which were formerly addressed through risky surgeries, by treating them as psychosomatic struggles that manifest as pain in the body. Myers understands many of these "mental issues" are in the tissues and that they can be solved by bodywork and the applied techniques of myo-fascial release. At the very least, he believes the techniques he gives should be a first line of treatment as opposed to invasive surgery or a lifelong dependency on pharmaceuticals, be they painkillers or psychiatric drugs.

Our injuries, large or small, have cumulative effects. Sometimes they are so subtle that even as they worsen, we remain unaware of them while our bodies become desensitized. Over time our bodies work themselves into psychosomatic knots which can show up as anything from depression to chronic pain, or limited range of motion to crippling emotional states. We must address these ailments before proceeding to power and stamina training. If we do not, then such training will only cause the body to work against itself and compound the situation, not unlike heavy weightlifting with a cramped or strained muscle. In the best-case scenario, we miss out on the training's maximum benefits and the optimal transformation we seek. In the worst-case scenario, which is inevitable in the long run if we do not pick up on our body's warning signs, then the result is serious damage.

Breath is our consistent tool for opening and closing various parts of our body. Voice extends the reach of our breath. It sets our molecular makeup into a state of vibration. Tones direct our voice's capabilities to focus on specific target areas with resonance. Working from the inside out, these tools are priceless, especially when combined with proper posture and movements. However, certain injuries put our bodies into such states that the effectiveness of breath, voice, posture, and movement as tools to heal ourselves become severely limited. Fortunately, the solutions are often as simple as the healing power of touch.

THE QUEEN OF DE-ARMORING
AND THE MAN IN THAILAND

My wife and I had just married. In the few years previous, I had been working for a horrendous employer in Norway to be closer to my, at the time, girlfriend, to save up money and begin my life with her in Denmark. In the end, the employer bankrupted the company and hid my employment records with an outstanding debt of 800.000 NOK owed to me.

Despite being cheated, I had managed to save enough money to get a little start, and my wife and I were happy. Maybe it was the winter, her new job, the long drive to work, or the unspoken social pressures of how one "should" lead a married life, but the day we married my wife's sex drive went flat. Somehow sex no longer was the celebration it once was. As her mentality around sex changed into a perfunctory act meant for making babies, so did her physical experience of it. In fact, her physical experience changed so much that sex even became painful. It was a challenging time for us. Fortunately, we had built our relationship on more than the physical, and we were dedicated to working through this trial.

At the pinnacle of this tribulation, my wife happened to find a tantra masseuse and bodyworker named Pernille Ørnsøe Knudsen. She lived about an hour and a half from us and could just squeeze us in for a session before she went on vacation. She was a blessing for us both. She spoke into our relationship and specifically, into my wife's struggles in a way that only another Danish woman could. She explained that many women she sees go through similar experiences. Equally important, Pernille recommended a tantric workshop for women on sisterhood, as well as a bodyworker by the name of Susanne Roursgaard.[3] Pernille could not speak highly enough of her skills and character and told us she would personally go to Susanne when in need of bodywork.

Susanne Roursgaard, or Sus as she is often called, is a former midwife but now works full time giving vaginal de-armorings as well as anal and cock de-armorings to men. A trained sexologist and couple's therapist, as well as a slew of other accreditations, she works not only with the physical body, but the psychological and energetic bodies as well. She has a knack for surfacing repressed physical and emotional pains as a means to help her clients release their past traumas. After attending the women's tantric workshop and there receiving a vaginal de-armoring from another woman, my wife's curiosity was peaked. She contacted Sus for a session. Eager to learn but still a little uncertain as to what to expect, she made the forty-five-minute drive feeling somewhat uneasy in her body.

To begin the session, Susanne took the better part of an hour to explain that many of her clients experienced a full range of emotional and physical reactions during a session and my wife should feel free to express and voice them if needed. Everything from anger, flailing legs and arms, laughter, crying, yelling, joy, etc., was normal. A formerly conservative and soft-spoken Dane, my wife was a bit skeptical that would be her need, but she was glad to know that Sus would be there for her if these reactions did arise. The experience for her was transformative to say the least. She was blown away by how much unknown stress, anger, and physical pain she had stored up and had been carrying around in her body. She booked a second session, after which I contacted Sus and requested that we share a dinner with her and her husband. Not only did I want to express my deepest gratitude for the work she had done on my wife, but I also wanted to communicate my desire to learn a "light touch" de-armoring technique from her *Gaia Method*. As she did not consider herself a mentor, my initial request was declined.

Still curious and hungry for knowledge, I decided to book a de-armoring with Sus so I could experience it myself. I figured any wisdom I picked up from her touch would only be an added benefit. I gained much. As good fortune would have it, some months later I was pleasantly surprised to find out that she was offering a one-day vaginal de-armoring course in Copenhagen. My wife insisted that I attend even though she couldn't due to prior obligations. She paired me up with another woman whom we had met the week prior at a small tantra gathering—this woman also wanted to attend the workshop, but was missing a partner. The knowledge, inspiration, and tactile abilities I gained from Sus's workshop birthed a calling within me that has only continued to blaze brighter and brighter to this very day. Immediately following the workshop, I knew I wanted more practice.

With my wife's amazing trust and full blessing, I de-armored another woman who was a professional bodyworker, colleague, and weekend host to Sus. The following day I de-armored yet another woman, a Swedish artist and former gymnast, whom my wife and I had met some weeks before. Finally returning home later that evening, I proceeded to de-armor my wife that night and again the following day. I did not stop there. I contacted our friends, who contacted their friends, and after their self-professed "wonderful" results, they in turn contacted their friends. I spoke with women I met on the street, at the gym, in women's groups, at dinner parties, and basically anyone who I sensed might be curious or in need.

Within a few months I had de-armored nearly fifty different women and had performed copious sessions on them as well as my wife. My very happy and now highly sexually responsive wife was reaping all the benefits, as my skills, techniques, and experience grew by leaps and bounds. With all the imprints I was receiving from each session, coupled with my past experience in the healing and martial arts, my sessions had become something of their own and incorporated hydration, breath, voice, trance, movement and many of the exercises you are receiving in this book.

As word got around, it was Sus who asked me for a session in exchange for whatever knowledge I would gain from her body and feedback. After the session, she wrote a big thank you to my wife where she readily acknowledged that what I was offering was both unique and beyond a basic de-armoring. She offered to help further hone my skills and suggested that I give a unique name to my session and techniques. Where Sus's skill set, touch, and specialty led clients through the deep healing of trauma releases, my touch unlocked the

Queen within them, awoke their femininity, and reconnected them to their own pleasure system.

The feedback from women was that my sessions were therapeutic, and helped them feel feminine, grounded yet weightless in their body, trusting, and an increased empathy and fluidity in navigating social relations and situations. They said it increased (or sometimes allowed for the first time) facility in achieving orgasm on their own or with a partner, as well as brought about a sense of white light and energy pulsing throughout and from their bodies. It quickly had become apparent that there seemed to be quite a demand for this work in Scandinavia. Many women confessed to having had feelings of being disconnected from their femininity, often accrediting it to cultural pressures and lacking the needed relief from their otherwise masculine roles and mode of operating both at work, in the gym and at home.

I began cold calling doctors, psychologists, sexologists, prostitutes, journalists, bodyworkers, and lawyers[4] to hear their professional perspective on the feedback I was receiving and the service I was offering. If I felt led to, then I would propose a trial session, which most readily accepted (over 95%).

One such call was to Signe Bentzen,[5] the renowned couple's therapist, former president of the Danish Sexology Union, and journalist. As a result of the phone call and session, she went on her show *Sexperterne* announcing to Denmark her high praises of the experience.

To gauge the response, I quickly had a very basic website made. Despite still being under construction and therefore consisting only of a three-question questionnaire, it received around 2,800 hits in two days. It was another telltale sign that there was a huge Danish demand from women seeking to facilitate embodied transformation.

I began to scour the internet and library for more pertinent information as I continued to further hone my skills. It had been a little shy of a year, and I had given away around 100 sessions, when my wife complained of some blocked energy in her stomach. I came across a fantastic video by a man from Thailand who was giving a seminar in Germany on abdominal massage, reflexology, and the body's meridians. He was demonstrating on himself as well as a woman and man. I followed his movements on myself and began to study various maps on the meridians, abdomen, and Chinese reflexology. Later that night I applied what I had learned on my wife, with great success. I incorporated the knowledge and teachings into my sessions by not only giving the preliminary full-body massage but by focusing on several trigger points in relation to the meridians in the abdominal and leg regions. I quickly noted a more facile release of tension when working on the vagina. In addition, I was able to provide results on a deep level for those women who wanted to get in closer touch with their femininity, but were themselves shy about a vaginal de-armoring session, or had a partner who was initially a little uncertain, too closed, or jealous about another touching their partner's sexual temple.

I spoke to a colleague and friend, who had received many sessions from me in return for her verbal as well as bodily feedback, Gry Dagmar Schødt Møberg.[6] Gry herself is a phenomenally eclectic therapist and bodyworker. She wields many traditional, as well as shamanistic, tools from around the world, and is currently working with the celebrity, business, and cultural leaders of Scandinavia to hone their leadership potential. She has a knack for knowing most everyone in the field of bodywork and told me the man was none other than Mantak Chia. Though I have never met him, his video sparked my interest, exploration, and discoveries with abdominal bodywork. I am grateful for that video, Sus and Gry's influence on my learning curve, calling, and this field of work.

WHEN MORE IS LESS

The most common mistake of bodyworkers, masseuses, and healers is to attempt to do or make something happen. Often, they focus too much attention on themselves or whatever technique they have decided in advance to apply. In turn they forget the most important rule of bodywork: **Work with the person, not against their body.** Before Gry's first session with me, she recounted a story of the first time that she received a vaginal de-armoring.

The young bodyworker, who was practicing on Gry, had just been to an introductory tantra workshop where he was introduced to a forceful (*hard touch*) de-armoring "technique." The rules of thumb were that if nothing seemed to happen then apply more force and pressure. If it hurt, then you were doing it correctly. If the receiver complained of pain, then tell them to process it. When he applied this philosophy, inevitably it became a battle between his body's force and hers. The result was that Gry, an untamed warrioress with Viking blood streaming through her veins, launched him across the room with a reactionary yet solid kick to the face. He had tried to resolve her vagina's resistance and blockage by jabbing his finger in with yet more pressure. I understood the story was didactic and for my benefit.

I let her know that I didn't think this would be the case with me. After all, I told her, I liked my face. I explained that she would be doing most of the work. The session turned out to be phenomenally successful. I learned a lot, and she titled me a wizard. Gry then began to spread the word about me. So, what made the difference between her first vaginal de-armoring session and the one with me? I believe that it was my intention.

As opposed to a set result, my intention was to hold masculine space for her feminine to emerge and to be an active guide if ever she became stuck or frustrated. As bodyworkers, therapists, and healers, we may hold all the keys, but as opposed to crafting solutions ahead of time it is the receiver who must present the door and lock before we begin to mold the key to help them open past their challenges. My greatest efforts and works are to invite the trust, confidence and courage of the recipient so I can accurately find, present, and guide them through overcoming that which binds them. This presupposes an adaptive interaction with well-set intentions, requiring an active receiver and a receptive actor on behalf of the client and bodyworker.

TUNING THE INSTRUMENT

My experience and belief is that the body of a healthy adult naturally enjoys and desires sex. The same as food, water, breath, and the need for community, sex is not an itch to scratch or superfluous luxury to be had. The nurturing of sexual energy is a healing, balancing, and rejuvenating need. To abstain from or neglect it can carry negative consequences. Regarding frequency and quantity, this of course varies according to appetite, age, and the ebb and flow of life. Furthermore, I do believe there are benefits and various reasons to sexually fast. It may be a fast from sex with others while maintaining your own self practice, or it may be refraining altogether from any sexual activity for periods of time. I would, however, disagree that the once a week, once a month, or even less frequent desire for sexual practice is a healthy norm but instead an indicator of a closed-down body. Similarly, the insatiable, consuming craving for indiscriminate sex can also be a sign of sexual malnourishment and addiction. An unblocked and open body physiologically responds to the potential for sex with increased blood circulation, hormone production, etc. However, as opposed to then needing to act upon an impulse, or shaming yourself over it, a balanced person is simply able to enjoy the arousal for its presence. They can then choose to act on the arousal or not. Like an instrument that is in tune, the body will resonate when another in-tune instrument is played in its proximity. If either instrument is out of tune, then the resonant effect is severely diminished, if not absent, and no music is shared. Just like a string instrument's tuning pegs need be turned upon occasion, the body's tissues from time to time must be touched into tune. This is not a prescriptive process of three turns up and four twists down, but an interactive one. The tuning must be done relative to the instrument's current state. As such, the instruments current state is only ever known by plucking its strings and listening.

You've learned your instruments notes in Exercises 5, *Resonant Voicing*. Now let's learn some technique for how to tune it with touch.

YOUR TECHNIQUE: THE ART OF SOFT TOUCH

Some people prefer a firm touch followed by a light one, others a light touch followed by firm. Some simply want it light and others always firm. However, especially when it comes to bodywork and healing, there seems to be a rather heated debate between certain schools of thought. Some adhere to the hard-pressure school of "no pain no gain." Others use the touch of "no touch," as in certain applications of Reiki. My experience is that the tighter, tenser, or more exhausted the instrument is, then the lighter the touch should be at first. The more tuned the instrument is, the more firmly you can play its strings. Whether it is hypertension or over-exhaustion, these are two sides of a closed or irresponsive state. A balanced, responsive body is termed "open." As Thomas

Meyers states in his YouTube video "Why Does Massage Hurt,"[7] he identifies three types of pain: Pain that enters the body, such as when we bump our head; pain that resides in the body, of which we are often unaware or have become accustomed to; and the pain of pain leaving the body . . . the last being the only form of "good pain."[5] It should be understood that even the lightest touch can be experienced as excruciating pain in a tense or injured person. However, a firm touch in the exact same place, on the same person once the tension is released, can catapult them into heights of ecstatic pleasure. Whether applied hard or soft, techniques are the tools of touch, and tools are only as good as that for which they were designed.

DE-ARMORING

Though there are many "de-armoring" rituals and practices the world around and dating back as far as people began using their hands to heal, the psychosomatic term "armoring" was coined by one of Freud's top students, Wilhelm Reich (*Character Analysis*, 1933). His insight was revolutionary in understanding that our body is part of our mind and that our muscular rigidities contain the history of their origin. By this I mean that muscular tensions set in as people's patterns for physical behavior form into bodily habits, such as posture, tone of voice, etc. Reich called this physical rigidity *armor* and the corresponding psychological state *character armor*. Reich would treat his patient's body posture with corrective braces and even, to Freud's great disapproval, push into their body's sore spots to affect change in their character.

Below are several techniques to use in the overall de-armoring process. They will be especially useful in addressing any of the trouble spots encountered in the breathing and voicing exercises.

EXERCISE 21: Trigger Point Touch

This exercise will teach you, the giver, an isolated touch technique about the importance of pressure and stillness. This is the opposite of what most people think of as massage, in which they employ kneading or other moving techniques. In addition, it will teach you person-specific patience, and attentiveness towards what the receiving body tells you. After all, it is their bodily needs which must take primacy over your own preconceived notions of rhythm and pace.

1. Make Contact

    a. This should be done lightly and with heightened awareness, so the receiver's body can establish trust with your touch.

    b. Slowly increase pressure until solid contact is made with the flesh of the receiver and then gently release until a pulse or current is felt under the finger.

    c. Gauge the reaction as either a sign of Tension, Exhaustion, or Openness, as detailed in the following step.

2. Reaction

a. Tension

- Signs of tension are a vocalized report or an expression of pain. Normally pain can be first noted in the outer corners of the eyes. They will wince and form crow's feet when subtle. A less subtle sign is a reactive jerk, or violent yelp in more extreme cases.

- When applying light touch to tension, be sure the recipient is continually breathing, and voicing with sound whatever it is that they are feeling. Give them permission so they know they do not need to hide the voicing of pain. Remind them as necessary. This is especially true for men. I have found that men are more likely to try and hide pain, but once permitted have much more to voice, as their pain tolerance is much lower than that of women.

b. Exhaustion

- Signs of exhaustion are a general numbness, expression of irritation marked by no response, or the look of fatigue, after which the body becomes squirmy and the person irritable and even snappy.

- When applying light touch to exhaustion, imagine bringing them back to life as you invigorate them. Alternate between quickly releasing and reestablishing the touch while very, very, very gradually increasing the intensity of release and then reestablishing touch. Beginning gently, and with a connection of trust between the giver and receiver, is important. The recipient should use their inhalation to push against your touch while voicing their sensations on the exhalation.

c. Openness

- Signs of openness are an overall relaxed face (especially around the jaw and eyes), facility in taking full, deep breaths, and ease in giving over the weight of their relaxed body into your touch.

- Once trust is established, it is like the perfect wave that does not overpower or crash a surfer. Follow their pleasure and build steadily towards their body's wants as you progressively take the lead. Note that building steadily does not mean doing "more" but instead continuing what you are already doing with more focus. As their pleasure begins to increase, they may desire more, more, and more pressure, but only do so in proportion to the established trust.

3. Application

a. Holding the tension points, have them breathe into your contact so that they control the pressure. Have them voice the tension with vibration in their vocal chords as they exhale, so that they own the release. Wait until you feel the tension melt under your touch, like cold butter into warm. If it does not melt at first, then continue elsewhere before returning.

EXERCISE 22: **Myofascial Release**

~~~~~~

This exercise will teach you about the importance of stretching the receiver's tissues on a microscopic level.

1. Contact

    a. With one hand, make the initial contact as with de-armoring. When solid contact is made, hold it.

    b. With your other hand, make the same solid contact at another point along the body's natural lines (i.e. the same meridian or myofascial train) and hold.

2. Stretch

    a. Gently stretch the two points in opposite directions and hold.

3. Twist

    a. While maintaining both the contact and stretch between the two points, gently twist one of the fingers without hurting the skin. The skin should not slip under your contact but visibly twist with your finger. Hold, and then gently twist the other finger in the opposite direction. Hold from one to five minutes, untwist, then release the stretch and finally relinquish contact before proceeding elsewhere.

EXERCISE 23: **Spacing**

This exercise will teach you the importance of creating space between muscles, as well as other bodily structures, for removing numbness and rigidity so as to return plasticity and range of motion to a tense body.

1. Make contact to the *linea semilunaris* with the blade of your hand or the side of a finger. The fingertips can still be used and are particularly good when progressing more deeply. However, you should be aware that they often can be too direct and forceful at the outset for the recipient's body to surrender into trust.

2. Have them push against your pressure with their inhalation and relax further each time with their exhalation.

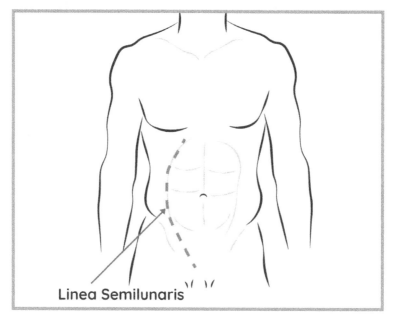

Diagram 14

3. With your contact, follow their exhalation deeper into their body. Use gentle wiggles and rocking motions to create more space between the muscles while continuing to progressively sink in deeper.

4. Continue until the needed space and depth is obtained for the body to feel open and free, showing signs as described in Exercise 23, step 2.c.

5. Repeat on the other side.

TROUBLE SPOTS

When practicing your belly breathing, voicing, and these three de-armoring techniques, you may note places in your body where discomfort or feelings of blockages continue to return or never quite leave. When dealing with these or other points, you may also notice that certain emotions continually surface, or colors come to mind. You should know that not all blockages are purely physical. The following exercises contain strategies for working with these trouble spots.

EXERCISE 24: Colors and Chakra Voicing

As shown in Diagram 1, each chakra has its own color as well as sound. This exercise will teach you a useful technique (passed on to me by my friend Henrik Frydendahl) for dealing with energetic blockages that trigger the visual or sense of colors.

1. Using Exercise 21, *Trigger Point Touch,* position your finger over the point of discomfort or blockage.

    a. You can also or simply place the Lao Gung point of your hand over the affected spot.

2. If a color is seen or comes to mind, then take your free hand and place it over the chakra of the corresponding color.

3. Visualize taking the color and blocked energy away from the trouble spot. Bring the colored energy up your arm over the trouble spot and cycle it through your other arm and back into the chakra.

4. In addition to Henrik's technique, I have found that the effect can be increased by using belly breathing and Exercise 5, *Resonant Voicing.*

    a. Pull up the blocked energy in your arm on the inhalation, returning it through the other arm to the corresponding chakra while voicing its specific tone on the exhalation.

    b. Use long deep breaths, filling up your lungs and belly to the maximum, then releasing the breath slowly and with as much vocal resonance as possible, until you have exhaled absolutely all remaining air. This can be loud. If you are not applying this technique to yourself, then the giver should time her or his breath with that of the recipient's, and both should voice together.

EXERCISE 25: Emotions and the Six Healing Sounds

As you may have noticed in breathing and voicing Exercises 1-7, as well as with the bodywork de-armoring techniques in Exercises 21-23, your system becomes activated as you are put in touch with it. Therefore, it is normal that these practices will cause certain emotions to surface. Sometimes they surface right away, during the exercise. Sometimes they creep up slowly, building over the next several days. At other times they can just suddenly pop up out of nowhere, several days after the exercise. For many years, Taoist medicinal practitioners have understood that our internal organs are not only linked to various other points on our bodies as described in reflexology, but are linked to our various emotional states as well. Furthermore, our internal organs, like our chakras, are affected by the resonance of various tones. The use of these tones and voicing allows us to bring balance to our internal organs and their corresponding emotional states.

If you notice that the trouble spot resides in the area of one of the particular organs or that the emotion that continues to arise is one listed below, then inhale deeply into the corresponding organ and voice the corresponding tone on the exhalation.[8]

1. Lungs
    a. Inhale courage, self-empowerment, determination, and confidence.
    b. Exhale your sadness and depression, emotional pain, and numbness while voicing the sound *hsssss*.
2. Kidney
    a. Inhale gentleness, calmness, serenity, and tranquility.
    b. Exhale your fears, apprehensions, and anxiety while voicing the sound *chooooo*.

3. Liver

    a. Inhale kindness, generosity, and gratuity.

    b. Exhale your rage and greed while voicing the sound *shhhhhh*.

4. Heart

    a. Inhale love, joy, playfulness, and compassion.

    b. Exhale your impatience, hastiness, and apathy while voicing the sound *haaaaa*.

5. Spleen

    a. Inhale openness, centeredness, faith, and optimism.

    b. Exhale imbalance, mistrust, and pessimism while voicing the sound *hoooooo*.

6. Triple Warmer (Your Brain, Heart, and Perineum)

    a. Inhale compassion.

    b. Exhale any excess heat from your brain, heart, and perineum while voicing the sound *sheeee*.

CHAPTER FOUR:

PLASTICITY, STAMINA AND POWER

YOUR PLASTICITY: THE WHITE LINE

In 2007, I visited Australia to give a weekend workshop in my role as a social coach with Charisma Arts. On a bus ride back from Bondi Beach, heading into downtown Sydney, I met a striking Danish woman with lavender eyes, built like a model. Sparked by our connection at that first meeting, she and I began a long-distance relationship and over the next several months, fell in love over written letters, SMS, and phone calls. She came to visit me at home in the U.S. and met my family before I began a nine-month fellowship program at Trinity Forum Academy on the Chesapeake Bay.

Searching for ways we could be together, I stumbled across an MA program in Cognitive Semiotics at the University of Aarhus close to where she lived in Denmark, and I enrolled. It was the ideal program to follow up both my time working with Charisma Arts and my BA in Linguistics from the University of Michigan. I had written my BA Honors Thesis on how language is used in cults to brainwash people—termed *coercive persuasion* in the field of psychology—and to create group dynamics run by fear. After such a dark theme, I found myself wanting to focus my studies at Aarhus on delving into studying the behavioral patterns of body language, speech, attachment psychologies, and neurochemical releases that most successfully lead to individuals sparking attraction amongst each other and coupling together.

Ironically, it was as I studied and wrote about the nuances of social relationships that for the first time in my life, I had a girlfriend cheat on me. She cheated several times, and while in the middle of the two-year program I ended the relationship. Frankly, I was crushed.

After a six-month dating hiatus, I decided to allow myself to jump back into the pool. From my ex-girlfriend and her family, I had learned a lot about the struggles people face when trying to pair bond and build lasting relationships after growing up in families with histories of rampant divorce. I also learned about the sexual stagnation and death of passion which come from depolarized relationships—by depolarized relationships, I am referring to where the dance of masculinity and femininity between partners becomes neutered, and how a history of one-night stands conditions avoidant attachment and infidelity. (You will find more information on avoidant attachment as well as the other attachment types in Chapter 7's section, *Background Check*.)

After the breakup, the conversations with my Danish university friends and experiences dating other Danish women only reinforced my observations. I cannot say that these relationship and attachment observations are unique to Denmark and Scandinavia at large, any more than they are to any culture with high divorce rates, the unsatisfying and misappropriated philosophical overspill of egalitarianism and modern feminism into the bedroom, and a reasonably high level of social acceptability with minimal levels of reproach for sexual libertinism and nights seasoned by the heavy consumption of alcohol. Yet there is an oddity I came across which seems somewhat pervasive in the sexual struggles of women raised and living in Scandinavia: namely the length of time and concentration required to reach orgasm. Not only had I begun to become aware of this from my own experiences, but from the many reports shared by my Norwegian, Swedish, and Danish friends of both genders.

I refer to this struggle as an oddity because, undoubtedly, Scandinavian women are some of the most generally fit, highly-educated, free, and beautiful women in the world. One would imagine that orgasms for them would be easily achieved and highly powerful, yet never have I encountered such a high percentage of women who were clitoral dependent for orgasms and, more importantly, who struggled to reach orgasmic release. I would have likely written off this observation as just chance and due to a small sampling, except for an unexpected twist in fate.

I was finishing my final year at Aarhus University and had learned upon entering the dating pool in Denmark that "dating," in the traditional sense, isn't exactly the norm. In fact, I was much more likely to terrify a woman with an offer of dinner, than with a random thirty-minute chat over coffee, a few drinks at the bar, and a direct invite home for no-strings-attached sex. It was not that I was particularly partial in any sense to traditional dinner-dating culture, but I found myself wanting to know the woman I was interacting with on a deeper level, and over a period of time, before becoming sexual with her. I had already concluded that I never wanted another long-distance relationship after my experience with my ex-girlfriend. Also, my fair share of "dating" experiences did not incline me to pursue a committed relationship with a Scandinavian. I'm not sure if the latter was solely *my* choice, or that of the women who didn't seem overly interested in anything more than just "having fun." Life always has the last laugh, however, and it is said, "Never say never."

Almost as soon as I had nearly sworn off Scandinavian women, I met a woman who would change my thinking. Thankfully, I was not so stubborn in my mindset that I let myself stand in the way of the opportunity and gift life placed before me. After nearly five years of a long-distance relationship with a magnificent and beautiful Danish woman, I married her. Never have I experienced such richness in dedication, responsibility, love, trust, and honesty as I have with her, nor have I learned so much about women.

As our social network joined and continued to grow, my initial observation on clitoral dependence in Scandinavia continued to be confirmed, and my curiosity grew. I asked further into how they had sex, what positions, if and how they reached orgasm, etc. At tantric gatherings I observed how they were having sex, how they breathed and moved. This led me to a second observation. The women's movements during intercourse seemed counter-intuitive to me, and somehow inhibitory for more profound orgasmic releases. The movement reminded me of something, but I could not quite put words to it. At first, I thought it might just be our university friends and the inability to put down one's guard and a need for control as games of dominance are common in one-night stands. However, the reports not only came from women who were having one-night stands—the experience seemed equally rampant among our friends who never had one-night stands, those with relatively little sexual experience, and even those well-versed and seasoned in tantric circles. Eventually it dawned on me. The movements and breathing postures the women were embodying as they became more sexually aroused were those typical to clitoral stimulation and specifically the use of vibrators . . . even if they were not touching their clitorises or had long thrown out their vibrators.

Looking for further insight into this geographic clitoral enigma, I found that many women were introduced to masturbation by their mothers or friends, yet were only made aware of how to reach orgasm on their clitoris. Later, when of age, they bought vibrators. Now this, in and of itself, may not be unique to Scandinavia. However, relative to the rest of the world, the lack of stigma around female masturbation and the extent of socio-cultural promotion for women to be sexually self-sufficient may be, I believe, unique to the area. In Scandinavia, vibrators are promoted as a tool for sexual self-sufficiency and the initial facility for quick orgasms has made them quite the alluring alternative to not only fingers but partners . . . and from them (their vibrators) so many Scandinavian women have had the majority of their sexual practice. I would be curious to run a world survey on the number of vibrators there are per female capita to make a usage density map and see where in the rankings Scandinavia lies. However, it's not just women who have been "conditioned" in ways that disallow the richer experiences of great sex. The prevalence of male masturbation for a quick release would also define the majority of men's sexual practices. It is a shame that as opposed to making most men last longer it causes them to reach orgasm prematurely. Now I am a tremendous advocate for sexual liberation and self-sufficiency, and I admire Scandinavia as a beacon and forerunner in this respect. Yet unfortunately, the dearth of information regarding the long-term numbing effects and the dependency vibrators create in users seems to be no less present in Scandinavia than in the rest of the world. So perhaps I found out the *why* for what so many of my friends and acquaintances were sharing. Maybe I didn't, but what both women and I were more interested in was the *how* . . . how to help women have more satisfying orgasms.

I began to take mental notes to describe the sexually inhibitory movements I was observing. My goal became to couple Scandinavia's relatively positive attitude around female masturbation and sexuality, with a solid "how-to" for overcoming clitoral dependence and exploring other types of orgasmic bliss.

This is what I observed: during the act of sex and when trying to force orgasm, I noticed that a woman's hips would rock to the front and remain positioned ever further and further forward, as the rate or intensity of the man's sexual penetration increased. The breath was exhaled, almost pushed out more and more forcefully. Eyes closed. The jaw became set and the vagina clenched. The mind focused less on the interaction and more towards a fantasy or ritualized pattern of behavior until, with the breath often held at the full exhale, the orgasm was finally forced into being. Many women have even told me of their need to turn over and face away into a pillow or have the lights off to avoid "distractions" from their partner. The movement, breathing, and mentality—an almost curling in on oneself—seemed to have a near synergistic effect in limiting the range of motion, sensation, interaction, and overall experience of sex. Furthermore, over time, this practice seemed to decrease plasticity and the sensational effects of sex. It was as if pleasure itself was being contained and localized, forced by will and therefore disallowed from expanding throughout the body. My experience with highly orgasmic women advised the opposite.

There is a rarely mentioned and rather trivialized fibrous, connective tissue running the length of your abdominal muscles and dividing them from left to right. Attached at the xyphoid process, it proceeds down and wraps around the belly button before fixing onto the pubic symphysis, which connects to the clitoris in women, and the penile erectile ligament in men. It is called the *linea alba* and means "white line" in Latin, due to its color. When you belly-breathe, this "white line" is naturally stretched. In traditional medical literature the *linea alba* is considered rather unimportant, as it has few nerves. It is even common to have it cut surgically in laparotomy procedures. With the advance of myofascial research, however, it is becoming known that sensation, emotions, and memories are stored in the tissues of myofascia. I have found the *linea alba* to be no exception, especially when it comes to plasticity and the full-body expansion of one's sexual pleasure and orgasm beyond the genitals.

BREATHE INTO AND VOICE YOUR VAGINA

With everything I learned, I began suggesting to women to move and breath in such a way that would stretch out their *linea alba* and myofascia of the pelvic/urogenital region. The suggestions developed into a series of catch phrases such as "Breathe into your vagina," "She needs air to think," "You're too much in your head—think with your vagina," "Let me hear from her," and "Give her voice." Quickly, these phrases became inside jokes as the women, often with a smirk on their face, would casually exaggerate their breath mid-conversation.

With the simple breathing, movement, and voicing techniques covered in Exercises 26 and 27 on the following pages, the women's struggles and clitoral dependence lessened. Furthermore, I noticed that these same techniques helped men who were experiencing little sensation during sex. Most interesting to me was that it also helped those women and men who felt victimized by peaking into orgasm too quickly . . . and yes, you read correctly that I wrote *women*. Albeit to a much lesser extent than men, I also have women tell me that they would regularly reach clitoral orgasm all too soon from little or no physical stimulation, sometimes before penetration, or even just from their partner's suggested approach. No, they did not consider themselves fortunate or lucky, since their body would then become too sensitive to engage in penetrative sex. Some even described a throbbing, nearly debilitating pain through their clitoris and the front side of their vaginal canal that inhibited them from foreplay and otherwise pleasing their man. In fact, a part of these women's understandable frustration is the fact that they are unable to speak about the issue, especially to their female friends who have sometimes become envious, and told them they were lucky and should appreciate their good fortune. Essentially, their friends told them to quit whining over what should be taken as a blessing.

So, whether you peak too early or struggle to orgasm at all, these techniques will help you increase your plasticity. In addition to Exercises 26 and 27, my clients can attest to the benefits of receiving an Imperial Session, as detailed in Chapter 5, *Optimal Sex*: Exercises 39 and 40.

TRANSFORMATIONAL VOICING (AKA DE-ARMORING WITH BREATH AND VOICE)

Not only are Exercises 26 and 27 helpful with the challenges of clitoral dependence, premature ejaculation and difficulty having orgasms, but they are a most natural way to de-armor and maintain a de-armored body with your own breath. They are especially designed to create plasticity in the urogenital area and open you up to full body orgasms.

EXERCISE 26: Genital Breathing (AKA De-armoring Breath)

This exercise isolates the factor of breath for de-armoring.

1. Begin seated at the zero point of Exercise 18, *The Clock*.
2. Inhale as you slowly arch your hips and lower back to the six o'clock position, while simultaneously arching your head, shoulders, and upper back backwards in the same direction as your hips.
3. Breathe into and fill your genitals, sacral chambers, belly, lungs, and throat so they expand to their maximum capacity.
4. On the inhalation, and when breathing into your genitals, use your breath to push out your pelvic floor muscles. Your perineum as well as your vaginal lips or penis should visibly swell and expand, as if blowing air out of your mouth with sealed lips.

5. With your xyphoid process and solar plexus lifting forward, feel your *linea alba* stretch.

6. Time the movement to reach its full arch as you reach the height of your inhalation.

7. Relax on the exhalation, allowing both the upper and lower body to return to the zero point. As you relax on the exhalation, relax your pelvic floor (PC) muscles so your perineum, as well as your vagina lips or penis, return to their neutral position without contracting any muscles.

8. With each inhalation, focus on expanding your genitals and belly further, creating more space and plasticity between and through the muscles and myofascia of your entire body. Be sure to do less with your muscles and more with your breath.

EXERCISE 27: **Genital Voicing (AKA De-armoring Voice)**

1. If you can, perform either of the next two items from behind, or from the front with both hands, then please do so. Otherwise, just use one hand:

    a. Women, cup your vagina from the base of your clitoris (not the tip of your clitoris, but the base where it goes under your pubic bone) to your anus with the Lao Gung point of your palm aligned over the entrance to your vaginal canal.

    b. Men, lifting your balls, cup from the base of your cock, where the underside of your sack connects to your body, all the way to your anus with the Lao Gung point of your palm aligned over your perineum.

2. Breathe in as detailed in steps 1-8 of *Genital Breathing*. Be sure to feel your genitals and perineum swell into your hand. Keep your thumb, index, and little finger extended. Women, you can insert your middle and/or ring finger into your vagina or anus. Men, you can do so into your anus. As you inhale, feel your vagina or anus swallow your fingers like a mouth. If exploring your vagina, then see how far you can lower your cervix with just your breath. With some practice, your cervix will be able to reach your fingers. If a man, then you can do the same to lower your prostate with your breath.

3. Relaxing on the exhalation, voice your root chakra long and steady, and with as much vibration and volume as possible. See if you can sense your voice's resonance in your hand.

4. Place your free hand on your second chakra and keep your other hand in place as you repeat steps 2 and 3 of this exercise, except voice your second chakra.

5. Keeping your right hand in place, continue moving your left hand up, one chakra at a time, voicing the chakra which corresponds to your left hand's placement and connecting it to your root via your right hand.

6. Once you are comfortable with the motion, breath, and voicing, repeat the exercise as you go through each of the sexual postures of Exercise 14, *Connecting the Postures*.

7. Focus on expanding throughout your body the sensation of kundalini energy and resonance from the vibration of your voice.

YOUR STAMINA: THE GREAT DEBATE

One debate in the world of neotantra[9] is in regard to stamina and whether one should train their PC muscles, or simply learn to relax them. The debate is over the false juxtaposition of training for strength, which works counter to relaxing the muscle. As with so many yoga positions in which one does train muscles, relaxation is simply a part of that training. In fact, when training for strength, even in weightlifting, you must learn to relax not only the muscles you are utilizing but even the ones you are not isolating in order to allow for the full range of motion to be achieved. One helps the other because relaxation aids in muscle recuperation after training, and proper training allows for deeper levels of relaxation. Whether one is training or relaxing, the breath is working and can be used to ensure that we "exercise" our full range of motion, strength, and maintenance of plasticity. I believe when most in the tantra world imagine training the PC muscles, they are thinking of common 'tense and release' or 'tense and hold' Kegel repetitions. The pitfall of such PC training is the build-up of tension if one does not also incorporate de-armoring into their routines. On the other side, I believe when those in the tantra world claim it is not enough simply to relax, they are speaking of literally doing nothing with their PC muscles. The pitfall for many beginners in "just relaxing" is that if they have never identified their PC muscles nor connected to their sexual system, then they will remain in a disconnected state.

As we develop our sexual practice, we must both train to strengthen and relax our PC muscles for maximal plasticity, as well as the guided allowance for the unhindered cycling of sexual energy and spread of orgasmic pleasure throughout the body. As one learns to better connect to his or her body during practices where there are higher levels of sexual energy, such as during intense intercourse, it is worth noting that for the well-trained individual less is more when contracting, expanding, or relaxing the PC muscles for the purpose of stamina. The same is experienced when transitioning from "external" martial arts to those termed "internal." The musculature used by advanced Dakinis and Dakas becomes more and more subtle, calling muscle control into action only when needed and only as much as needed. The PC muscles are neither overly relaxed where the energy and semen simply spills out, yet neither are they tense, creating energetic blockage and unintended build-up. Instead, the body takes on peaceful yet dynamic postures to wield its energy in the form of either *Cycling* or *Charging*. (I detail what is meant by these two terms in Exercise 29, 32, and 33)

THE MICRO ORBIT

Most people think of stamina as simply the ability to maintain a state of erection or wetness, but stamina is much more than that. In fact, true sexual stamina, just like breathing, is an ongoing process that most only consider when engaged in an overly sexual act, such as arousal, masturbation, or intercourse.

However, like ultra-marathon runners, iron men, Tour de France cyclists, or any practitioners of endurance disciplines will tell you, "The race starts long before the performance." In regard to sex, stamina is the ability to keep your sexual energy moving and not to become stagnant, built up, or trapped in one place. This is referred to as *Cycling* energy.

The track upon which our sexual energy cycles throughout our body is commonly referred to as the *Micro Orbit.* We can direct it with our breath and consciousness, aided by posture and movement. With our inhalation we draw in energy and project it out with our exhalation. By contracting our PC muscles we concentrate the energy, and by pushing the PC muscles out we expand the energy.

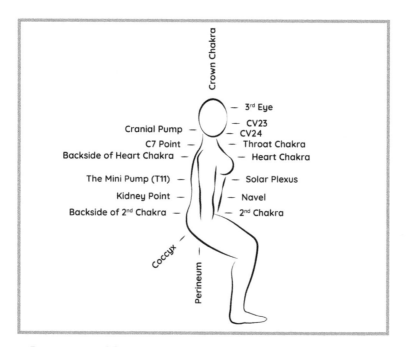

Diagram 15: The Micro Orbit and Energy Points

EXERCISE 28: **Pre-Cycling**

〜〜〜〜〜〜〜〜〜〜〜〜〜〜〜〜〜〜〜〜〜〜〜〜〜〜〜

Pre-cycling is simply an exercise to put you in touch with each of the main chakra points that run down your front and back centerline. The goal is to learn how to direct your energy up and then back down your spine, so that you are able to cycle it through your body's points along its microcosm, as shown in Diagram 15.

1. From the zero point of Exercise 18, *The Clock,* inhale as you expand your PC muscles and bring your body to the six o'clock position.

2. Feel your energy move up to your tail bone.

3. Exhale as you contract your PC muscles and bring your body back to the neutral position.

4. Feel your energy return to your perineum.

5. Start from your root chakra and continue this process of raising and lowering your energy. With each inhalation, bring the energy up your tail bone and spine by focusing one point higher on your micro orbit than with the previous breath (shown in Diagram 16) before returning it with the exhaled breath back the way it came to your perineum.

6. Continue inhaling your way up your spine one point at a time until you have passed your crown and reached your third eye. When you reach your third eye, allow the energy to cascade down your front side to your perineum as you exhale and contract your PC muscles.

EXERCISE 29: **Cycling**

This is simply putting together what you learned in pre-cycling for one smooth continual flow of energy.

1. From the zero point of Exercise 18, *The Clock,* inhale as you expand your PC muscles and bring your body to the six o'clock position.

2. This time, feel your energy move up through your tail bone all the way to your third eye.

3. Exhale as you contract your PC muscles and bring your body back to the neutral position.

4. Feel your energy flow down your front side and return to your perineum.

5. This is one cycle. Continue for nine cycles or until your energetic track becomes warm and tingly.

6. As you learn to navigate your inner energy track, allow yourself to become passively conscious of it so you are continually Cycling your energy throughout the day. Your movements will gradually become minimal as you primarily use your breath and consciousness.

ADDITIONAL TIPS FOR STAMINA

You can practice Exercises 28 and 29 during self-masturbation and sex with a partner to garner stamina by sensitizing your body, and giving you control over premature peak orgasms. However, here are a few additional tips for increased stamina that I discovered along the way to recovery from a rather debilitating urethral injury I discuss in Chapter 6: *Tools*. All three tips ensure that the body is in its most plastic state and can cycle sexual energy.

STAMINA TIP #1

Be well hydrated. By this I mean your urine should be rather clear. Don't be afraid to take pee breaks as needed when having a play date, and empty your bladder before intercourse or playing with your genitals as it not only clears the presence of bacteria from your urethral opening, but it gives the added benefit of letting both parties know that when The Queen begins to squirt (female ejaculate), she is not peeing.

STAMINA TIP #2

If you eat before sex, then choose light meals such as soups, vegetables, fruits, and purees. Waiting to eat after sex is best. You will be hungrier. The food will taste better, and your body will be primed and ready to absorb its full nutritional value.

STAMINA TIP #3

If engaging in intense exercise, then note that tension—and especially the buildup of lactic acid in the abdominal walls and urogenital area—will inhibit your plasticity. In turn, your ability to spread sexual energy and pleasure throughout your body will be diminished. This is particularly true of crunches and sit-ups as they compress the *linea alba*. Being especially fond of these abdominal exercises myself, I am not advocating forgoing them, but instead supplementing them with the following exercises.

SUCKING UP THE GUT

In our culture's eternal quest for the ultimate six-pack abs, many of us engage in all kinds of crunches and sit-ups in their numerous forms and variations. We are quick to neglect the transverse abdominal muscle, excepting of course that quintessential moment when we are walking down the beach, pass Mr. or Ms. Hotness, and suck up our gut. This action of course is rather a bit too little and much too late to leave the impression for which we hope. Considering the hours we sit on the couch or behind a desk, we inevitably fall victim to "furniture disease." Furniture disease is the widespread affliction of where your "chest" falls into your "drawers" . . . this is actually a favorite joke of my father's and I could not help but insert it. Excuse the pun.

Even bodybuilders, with their chiseled, gladiator build often have a gut when they are not flexing their abs. Fortunately the means to reverse this are rather simple. However, I must warn you the exercise is not "pain free." I came up with it after the urethral injury made me acutely sensitive to any tension in my abdomen, urogenital zone and especially in my *linea alba* between my belly button and pubic bone. While strengthening the transverse abdominal muscle, this exercise is especially good at stretching out everything from the top of the *linea alba* down to the penile/clitoral suspensory ligament. It is also great at reversing the compressed tension from all the abdominal exercises I enjoy so much.

EXERCISE 30: **Abdominal Dives**

1. Find a small throw pillow or fold a towel so that when you sit on it, you are elevated approximately 10-15 centimeters (4-5 inches) off the floor. When you lay back, the cushion should support you only as far back as your sacrum.

2. Lay back with your arms extended as if doing a reverse dive like the Olympic backstroke swimmers perform when launching into the pool.

3. From this extended position inhale and suck up your gut, creating as much space as possible between the lowest point of your abs and your pubic bone.

4. Remaining flat, and angled slightly down and towards the floor with your abs pulled up, exhale fully as you bring your arms to your shoulders.

5. Then, inhale sharply and fully as you pull up your stomach and explode out with your arms, diving down and back towards the floor. That is one repetition.

6. Reset to step 4 and continue repeating.

7. Try starting out with five sets of five repetitions. Workup to five sets of 10. When you can reach 50 repetitions in two sets of 25, then go back to 10 sets of 10 repetitions until you can reach 100 repetitions in two sets of 50.

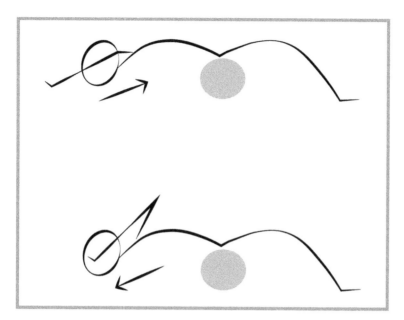

Diagram 16: Performing the Abdominal Dive

8. This exercise will require a lot of lower back strength. Go slow and take your time, especially if you have a bad back. If it is too intense, then you can bend your knees to 90 degrees or just hold the extended position while using your breath to pull up your abdomen and *linea alba*. Otherwise, simply skip this exercise until you have built up your lower back strength and focus on Exercise 31.

THE GURU OF BALI, ALWAYS BREATHING, ALWAYS MOVING

My wife had just finished an intensive two-week work trip. After instructing and updating communication protocols in her company's China, Thailand, and Indonesian offices, she was able to stay in South East Asia for a ten-day vacation. Taking advantage of this fantastic opportunity, she decided to surprise me by buying us both tickets to Bali. I would fly from Denmark and meet her there. With an ever-growing interest in yoga, she also booked us a seven-day stay at Guru Ketut's Om Ham Resort and Retreat where there were yoga courses twice a day, as well as many other activities, with food and spa treatments included. Located twenty minutes outside Ubud, Bali, at the base of the mountains and surrounded by picturesque rice paddies, the entire establishment was designed according to the instructions of Guru Ketut. Even the style of yoga was his own, and Guru Ketut, with the assistance of his pupils, led the daily Kundalini Tantra Yoga sessions. I can still hear the cat-like man, light in build and full of joy, calling out constant reminders as we participants strained to maintain what at first seemed like impossible positions: "Smile. Smile . . . always, breathing . . . always moving."

The sessions were active yet consciously focused, in that they required a fair bit of proprioception as the instructors continually corrected our posture, breathing, and the expressions on our faces into smiles. My wife and I gained many gems of knowledge and are so grateful for the opportunity to have practiced there.

The following is one of those gems, which I found relevant to the removal of tension in the abdominal walls, and to stretch out the *linea alba* for Cycling sexual energy and avoiding premature orgasmic peaking. Guru Ketut recommended it to massage your internal organs.

EXERCISE 31:

The Ketut Tummy Tuck and Urogenital Stretch

1. In a bent Horse Stance, where your chest is resting on your thighs, exhale all air from your stomach and lungs.

2. From your solar plexus to your pubic bone and under your ribs, pull up your abdominal wall and all internal organs within.

3. Stand up, bring your hips and chest to the six o'clock position so your *linea alba* is extended to the maximum while pulling up your perineum.

4. Feel your kidney, pulling up and stretching your urethral tubes so they tug at your ovaries/testicles.

   a. I recommend practicing this technique in an unaroused state. At step 3 you can use your hands to scoop up and

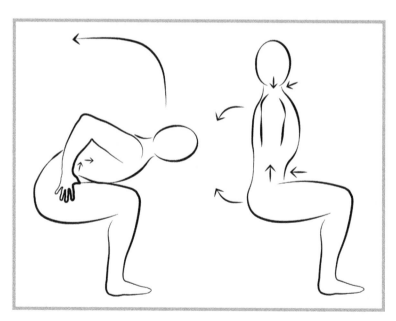

Diagram 17: Performing the Ketut Tummy Tuck

into your solar plexus to aid in pulling up your stomach. In addition, use the blade side of your hand (the outside of your palm from your little finger down to your wrist) to create space along the stomach meridian, as shown in Diagram 14 of Exercise 23: *Spacing.* This will aid to further pull up the lower region of your abdominal wall, as well as your urogenital organs, and ameliorate the circulation of your sexual energy.

b. After practicing in an unaroused state, incorporate this exercise into your solo masturbation and sex practice. It is most helpful in the case of emergencies where your energy gets stuck in your genitals and you are about to peak. Right before reaching "the point of no return," perform this movement and cycle the energy up from your perineum to your tail bone, sacrum, spine and into your micro orbit.

YOUR POWER: CHARGING THE BATTERIES

God works in mysterious ways. My wife and I were on our way back from the most excellent ten-day vacation in Bali at Guru Ketut's Om Ham Yoga Retreat. We were flying home to Denmark with a brief stop in Singapore and an all too brief layover for our connecting flight in Amsterdam's Schiphol Airport back to Denmark. I had been mentioning to my wife how great the yoga retreat was and that I would like to study Qi Gong. Little did I know that I would not have to wait so long for my Qi Gong introduction.

Schiphol was doing a passport check on exiting the plane,

which concerned my wife and I as we only had forty minutes to reach our final connecting flight. However, as it turned out, they were looking for me . . .

You can imagine my surprise, confusion and extreme frustration when I found out that Interpol had an arrest warrant out for me from Spain—with no further information. I can still remember the look of disbelief on my wife's face when I kissed her goodbye and told her to get on the flight back to Denmark.

Hours later, I was told that I was wanted for suspicion of fraud and the transportation of fraudulent documents! Several hours beyond that discovery, I found out that the warrant went back to a deal gone bad nearly six years in the past between a former employer and another company's boss. To top it off, the other company's boss had somehow put me in the middle and made me culpable to take the blame as the author of a scam he had tried to pull off. The reality sunk in that, one way or another, and without ever having been notified at my home address, Interpol would have its way and I would be going to Spain after however long the process of transfer would take in Holland. This most definitely did not fit into my life plan or jade egg and dearmouring business launch. The question, "God, why am I here?" played over and over again in my head like a scratched CD. I turned to prayer, meditation and training in the small airport holding cell. After being in isolation and then moved to several other detention centers, Holland finally decided on one where I would stay until being sent to Spain. Given my irregular training and sleeping hours

I was holding to the thought that having a roommate didn't seem like a good idea, and I prayed to have a room of my own. As usual, God had a bigger plan: I got a roommate. Within five minutes of conversation I found out he was a German Tai Chi and Qi Gong teacher who had suffered the misfortune of driving to Amsterdam with the wrong carpooler who had an unknown penchant for pick pocketing. When they arrived in the city, she stole a camera from a tourist and placed it on my roommate's person. He was barely able to communicate in English and not at all in Dutch to explain to the undercover officer what happened. He was simply taken in with the carpooler and sentenced for guilt by association. I hoped that a similar fate was not awaiting me in Spain.*

Though I didn't speak German nor he much English, we managed to communicate and become friends. Deciding to make the best of a tough situation, we exchanged our knowledge and practices.

The first two practices he taught me were the following exercises. They are gentle, yet an excellent start for charging your energetic batteries. A few details have been emphasized for the purposes of this book. Remember that all styles of training are one in that they deal with the human body. However, due to our intentions we use a technique in one way, while with another intention we would have used it in yet another way to best serve the moment's particular purpose. As this section is dedicated to power, let us first begin by identifying five of our

---

* To find out how this ended follow the link to the interview episode 11: http://optimalsexlife.com/interviewsemail

body 's main kidney points for drawing in and projecting out chi before proceeding to charging our sexual batteries. The kidneys are where the chi we were born with is stored, and they are considered by Taoist medicinal healers to be essential for working with your chi.

KIDNEY POINTS

These are the points to identify as we begin learning to charge our entire body with chi before proceeding to focus specifically on our sexual organs.

LAO GUNG

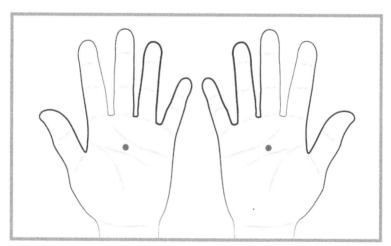

Refer to Diagram 2: Open Palms with Lao Gung Points

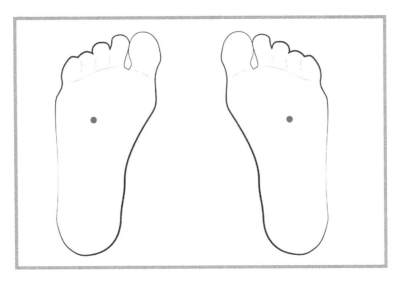

Diagram 18: Kidney Points under The Feet

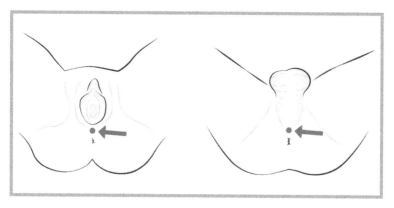

Diagram 19: The Location of Perineum on the Man and Woman Respectively

Now that we have identified the points we will be working with, let's begin to charge our entire body with chi before proceeding to focus specifically on our sexual organs.

EXERCISE 32: **Earth Charging**

This exercise draws energy from the earth and develops balance on and through your feet.

1. Inhaling, pull up from your perineum while scooping up energy from the earth. The hands stay close to the body with palms facing up towards the sky and thumbs away from the body. Move with your breath, keeping your arms and shoulders relaxed as you reach the level of your third eye.

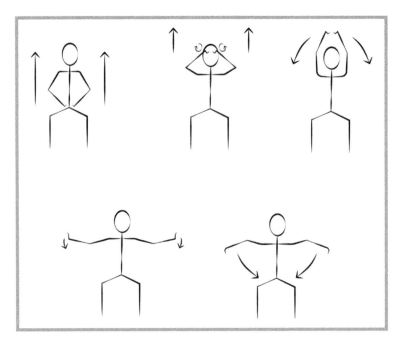

Diagram 20: Performing Earth Charging

2. At the level of your third eye, the palms flip over and away from your head as you begin to exhale. Relax your perineum. Moving with your breath, let your exhalation last until your hands reach the starting point.

3. As your hands return to the starting point, pull up your perineum and inhale as you begin anew.

4. Repeat nine or more times until your body feels warm and tingly.

EXERCISE 33: **Sky Charging**

1. Inhaling, pull up your perineum while scooping energy from the sky. Your hands should move with your breath, and keep your arms and shoulders relaxed as you reach the uppermost point where your hands join.

2. Exhaling, relax your perineum and while keeping your hands close to your body; lower your hands while you exhale, packing sky energy into your body. Reach the lowest point as the exhalation finishes.

3. As the palms turn up, begin your inhalation and pull up on your perineum as you return to the starting point.

4. Repeat nine or more times until your body feels warm and tingly.

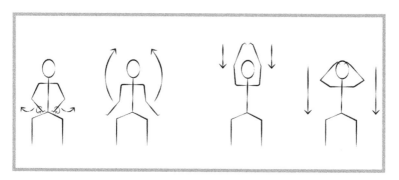

Diagram 21: Performing Sky Charging

SACRED CHAMBER CHARGING

Sus (Roursgaard) was giving another trauma release/vaginal de-armoring workshop for couples and she asked me to be her assistant, along with a few others. The vagina model for demonstrating her trauma release Gaia Technique was the Swedish Dakini Sanna Sanita. In addition to her impetus to share her talents with the world professionally, she has a big, loving heart on a personal level of which my wife and I have had the pleasure to come to know. At the time, I had never met her before, but while Sus was lecturing on theory, I could see by the way Sanna was sitting that her neck, hips and shoulders were carrying tension. Little did I know that she was in the middle of giving her own European tantra tour, and after all the flights, hotel hopping, and work, she needed a massage. I sat behind her, offered her a massage, and she gratefully accepted. Curious about my vaginal de-armoring sessions and in need of some bodywork, she invited me to Sweden. I worked on her the following weekend before she flew off to Berlin to continue her tour. After her return from Berlin, she had one final workshop in Copenhagen before ending her tour. The theme was breath work and full body orgasms. Sanna creates intensive, high energy workshops.

Desiring more bodywork for herself and help with the participants, she invited me to be an assistant. Her workshop was a smashing success. I was particularly intrigued by her breathing techniques where she guided participants on how to self-induce full-body orgasms. The techniques were like those I had been given for garnering power in my martial arts trainings. In fact, it was only the intention that was shifted. Instead of being martial, the intention was sexual. Later, I came across a brief, yet similar exercise in Saida Desilets's book, *Emergence of the Sensual Woman*, called Kundalini Breathing. The exercise I introduce below is for drawing in and projecting out your sexual power from your second chakra for the purposes of Charging your own self or someone else.

EXERCISE 34: **Kundalini Breathing**

This exercise is the gateway to experiencing what some refer to as breath or energy orgasms, when your whole body begins to buzz and eventually explode with waves of pleasure. The effect builds with the intensity and length at which you perform it.

1. Start in the neutral position from Exercise 18, *The Clock.*
2. Inhale fully, filling up your lungs completely while you contract your perineum and pull up your abdominal wall and internal organs as in Exercise 31, *The Ketut Tummy Tuck and Urogenital Stretch.*
    a. However, unlike the Ketut Tummy Tuck where you rock your hips backwards into the six o'clock position, rock your hips forward into the twelve o'clock position as you inhale.
3. Exhale and return to the neutral position.
4. Now inhale sharply, performing a series of quick inhalations each

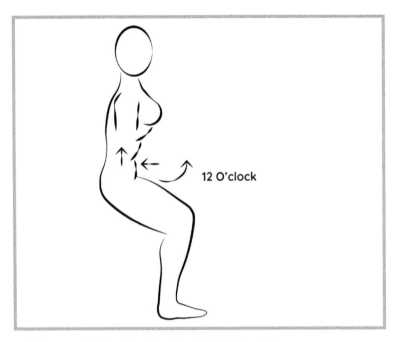

12 O'clock

Diagram 22: Performing Kundalini Breathing

time, progressively filling up your lungs more and more. Try to reach maximum lung capacity with the ninth inhalation.

5. With each of the nine rapid intakes of air, rock your hips further forward into the twelve o'clock position while progressively contracting your perineum and pulling up your abdominal wall and internal organs more tightly.

   a. Feel yourself filling up with and drawing in more energy to your Sacred Chamber (second chakra) through each of your Kidney Points, as shown in Diagram 2, 18, and 19.

6. In between the nine rapid intakes, do not exhale nor allow your hips to fully return to the neutral position or your perineum and abdominal walls to fully relax.

7. When you reach full lung capacity, hold both your breath and the

pull on your perineum, abdominal walls, and internal organs to continue drawing in energy to your Sacred Chamber.

    a. Hold for three or nine seconds if you are able to do so and of course taking care not to faint.

- You can use this to absorb energy from your environment, charging yourself from such sources as the earth, air, sun, and moon.
- If connected to another person, such as during sex or when de-armoring, you can use this to draw in their energy from the point of contact as well as the environment, to either charge yourself or unblock their flow.

8. Exhale fully, contracting and flexing your abs as you lower your abdominal walls, and internal organs while maintaining the contraction of your perineum and your hips in the twelve o'clock position.

    a. On the exhale, breathe out steadily yet forcefully over the space of three seconds, projecting the stored energy in your Sacred Chamber and out of the kidney point(s) of your choosing.

    b. If connected to another person, such as during sex or when de-armoring, you can use this to charge them from your own energy, from energy you absorbed from the environment, or to return what you just absorbed from them on the inhalation previously in step 7.

    c. If not connected to another person, you can simply return the energy to your environment. Your body will keep what is needed and return what is not.

9. Continue for as long as you enjoy, and take note how your overall stamina increases.

THE LEAST INFAMOUS ADDICTION

I remember my grandfather, an Air Force pilot and veteran lieutenant colonel from World War II, telling me how when he was in high school they had a sex education course in which each student was given a book. In this book was a section on masturbation, where the text gave dire warnings against such physical activity.

Two pictures he recollected most vividly were, first, a photo of two hands with hairy palms and, second, a picture of a man's face grotesquely covered in wrinkles. It was stated with "scientific certainty" that these misfortunes, as well as a premature death, awaited adolescent males who partook in masturbation. Being a man with a sense of humor and an absurd verbal filter, my grandfather recounted to me the schoolyard rhyme that he and his friends would sing in response to the book:

I don't care if I do die, do die!
I just want to make the juice fly, juice fly!

What must have been about sixty years after my grandfather's time, my fifth-grade sex education course gave a different "scientific" conclusion. Masturbation had become not only a healthy practice, but one that was recommended to us young boys. Oddly enough, I knew the word masturbation, but never really put any thought into how one would go about performing the act. Apparently, the absence of detail as to how one should or shouldn't masturbate had not changed in sixty years, and was one of the similarities that both educations shared. I imagine it has remained the same to this day.

I first ejaculated at the age of nineteen, after having received a blow job from an underwear model in a funhouse maze full of tunnels and slides. I remember feeling that although I enjoyed her gift, I didn't care for the ejaculation. Somehow it lowered my energy and made me feel down. I found a book at Borders Bookstore titled *The Multiorgasmic Man*, and thought it might provide instruction for a more interesting and alternative experience from the one in the maze. I had never had sex, but thought I might as well begin to teach myself the art of receiving and giving pleasure. I reasoned that when the time came for me to marry and please my wife, I would be ready.

As a devout Christian and the son of a preacher man and missionary parents, premarital sex was not on my "to-do list," so I spent my free time during my nineteenth summer reading about and practicing various masturbation exercises. I learned ejaculatory control, how to cycle my sexual energy, and how to build stamina and spread orgasmic sensations throughout my body.

It wasn't until two years later, at the ripe age of nearly twenty-one, that I first "lost" my virginity. I hardly "lost" it however. I was with the head cheerleader of a local university in the back seat of her convertible on a full moon night, and in the middle of an Indiana cornfield. There was some low hanging fog on the roads, and after some steamy kissing she said she wanted me inside her. I told her "no," as I felt sex was something that I wanted to be the one to initiate for my first time.

After having further aroused her with my hands I told her that now I wanted her. If anything, it was more of a "giving" then a "losing," yet unlike my training where I could last for hours, my first time having sex did not last as long . . . hahaha! For the rest of the summer we enjoyed training by practicing.

Eventually the relationship ended, but when I returned to university many of my once strictly-platonic female friends began to relate differently to me. So, I continued learning, but never really developed a particular liking for ejaculation. When I had sex for hours, me and my partner's energy would soar, leaving our bodies buzzing with orgasms and both feeling sexually nourished and satisfied. Looking back, I have also realized that I never really focused much on the clitoris. The women in my life were enjoying multiple orgasms from intercourse and didn't seem too interested in clitoral orgasms. Both the near absence of clitoral stimulation and ejaculation were never things I considered much of at the time. I simply thought that was how sex was for everyone. It wasn't until several years later that I noticed the standard of "good sex" was much lower than that to which I had become accustomed.

In the summer of my twenty-fourth year, I had to relieve my bladder just like any other time. However, when I went to the bathroom something that felt like a glass shard cut me right where the bladder connects to the urethra and became lodged. It stopped my urinary stream, but my bladder was still full. In an attempt to empty my bladder and evacuate whatever was stopping my stream, I forced myself to continue to pee, but instead of a regular urinary stream, red flowed out.

Three more times, whatever was inside became stuck, cutting me each time it dislodged, before finally passing out of my system. The toilet water had become a dark red. I never saw what was the culprit of this assault on my penis. All I knew was I felt there was something still stuck, and for the next five years I couldn't get a full erection without the head of my penis becoming swollen and semen simply spilling out. As you can imagine, this was painful and extremely frustrating. The doctors could give no explanation, and for the first year I basically forewent masturbatory practice and having sex. The following four years after that, I used trance states to regulate my pleasure and erection levels. I could feel that my sexual stamina and power was severely diminished, yet the women were still raving about the sex. I could feel that, even though they did not seem aware of or at least bothered about it, the heights of their sexual ecstatic potential had not been reached. It was then when I realized that the bar of what the status quo considers "sexual fulfillment" was quite low, and far less than their true potential.

During this time, I began to ejaculate more frequently while I tried to navigate my injury. As I did, I became aware that I, too, was no longer accessing the elevated levels of orgasmic pleasure I once had when I was not ejaculating. I'll share more about how I healed and regained access to these higher levels of orgasmic pleasure in Chapter 6: *Tools*.

I also began to further my manual and oral techniques, giving more attention to the clitoris, which led me to a second realization. The more frequently women had clitoral orgasms, the less capable they were of experiencing deeper, multiple, or full-bodied orgasms. It wasn't until attending a tantra seminar that I first heard someone else put my suspicions into words. They referred to the ejaculatory orgasms of men and the clitoral orgasms of women as "peak orgasms" and identified them as both desensitizing and inhibitory towards reaching our fully developed orgasmic potential.

People had always found me weird for not being fond of or not having the goal to ejaculate. It even made some women insecure, afraid they had not pleased me until I would explain to them that I could and preferred to orgasm without ejaculation.

When speaking with dedicated female clitoral advocates and male masturbators, I am often scoffed at and considered a lunatic when I suggest forgoing clitoral stimulation or male ejaculation for a time. The two most common reactions I hear are something to the effect of, "What would be the point of sex?" and "How would I ever relieve my sexual tension?" Almost unanimously, whether the person is an adept and attentive lover, or someone who considers sex as an itch to scratch, be they man or woman, the thought of abstaining from the peak orgasm over the course of one night of sex is met by serious resistance.

Most people can imagine postponing peaking so the other person will first reach their pleasure, but once that is obtained they want "theirs." You can read more about this in the section "Break the Routine: The Race and the Chase." in Chapter 5.

The widespread inability and severe resistance to even considering temporarily setting aside a type of pleasure for trying out something, which promises so much more, leads me to beg the question "Is it possible that the peak orgasm is the world's most unrecognized addiction?" I find people much more willing to skip meals, forgo food for a detox, spiritually fast, or completely cut out having sexual activity, than to consider having sex for a week while abstaining from peaking.

My personal experience is that from around fourteen days after a full ejaculatory release, the effect I have on women during sex is drastically different. The sexual energy and orgasmic experience they have is many times multiplied, even from partial penetration and without the use of friction. My penis, as opposed to getting hard from my desire, functions more like a magnet or tuning fork, responding only when the woman's vagina is open and emanating her resonant pull. From fourteen days and onward, I find that I am more influential in general and that women are specially drawn to initiate communication and to relate to me from a deeply feminine stance.

When de-armoring a woman I can sense by the tension in her clitoris if she has recently peaked or regularly peaks. The women who have not peaked for several months or more normally have soft clitorises, nearly as soft to the touch as the inner labia. After my sessions, many women also report feeling extreme amounts of sexual energy flowing through their body. The difference between those who report a continual flow of grounded sensuality and sexual charge for a day, versus those who feel sexual energy for several days or beyond a week, by in large depends on when they have their next peak orgasm. The flow of energy tends to subside not long after their next clitoral orgasm, where they focus on the tip and especially in conjunction with a vibrator.

Interestingly, those who do choose to climax on their clitoral head report that what normally could take them twenty or more minutes of concentration and hard work with their vibrators, fingers, or showerhead is instead easily achieved within a fraction of the time . . . sometimes less than a minute.

EXERCISE 35: The 21-Day Fast (Peak Orgasm Fasting)

Orgasm will have you either release and temporarily lose pleasure, or absorb, and gradually build it. This exercise will help you break the habit of releasing and diminishing pleasure, which is followed by a refractory or oversensitive period. This is the result of cumming with male ejaculation or by overstimulating the external tip of the clitoral head.

1. Continue your sexual practice, whether solo or with a partner, but for twenty-one days forgo peaking, as this is the standard time for overcoming an addiction.
2. Note if you experience any of the benefits mentioned.
3. Be sure to de-armor regularly, as the increase in energy will need to be cycled. Some people report feeling agitated, restless, and struggle to fall asleep, which is why I highly recommend remaining sexually active. This should subside after three days to a week as the body adjusts to the higher level of sexual energy.

a. I have included this chapter of power and stamina after the chapters covering breath, voice, posture, movement, touch, and technique, as the buildup of power in a blocked or ineffective system only exaggerates one's blocks and ineffectiveness. On the contrary, power in an open and effective system only begets more openness and effectiveness.

b. Taoist practices say it takes three months to recharge a fully emptied system, after which peaking once every fifteen days is not problematic. There is however much discrepancy over this, as some say it depends on age, some that one should never peak regardless of age, and others advocate peaking only once every one hundred sexual encounters.

  • I personally base my decisions on my penis' responsiveness to my wife's open vagina. Most importantly, have fun with your partner, avoid the trap of shaming yourself if you do peak, and seek out help if you really are struggling to enjoy sex due to premature peaking or a lack of sensation in your genitals.

EXERCISE 36: **Pre-Charging**

Pre-charging, like Pre-cycling, also puts you in touch with each of the main chakras along your front and back side. However, instead of moving your energy up and back down your spine by expanding your PC muscle you will be directing the flow of energy by contracting your PC muscle to initially move it up and back down your front side.

1. From the zero point of Exercise 18, *The Clock,* inhale as you contract your PC muscle, and bring your body to the twelve o'clock position.

2. Feel your energy move up to your sacred chamber (second chakra).

3. Exhale as you expand your PC muscle and bring your body back to the neutral position.

4. Feel your energy return to your perineum.

5. Continue this process of raising and lowering your energy. With each inhalation bring the energy up your front side one point higher on your micro orbit before returning it with the exhaled breath back the way it came, all the way to your perineum.

6. Continue inhaling your way up through your sacred chamber (second chakra), one point at a time, until you have reached the point at the base of your skull. When you reach this point, allow the energy to cascade down your backside to your perineum as you exhale and expand your perineum.

7. Try reversing the direction of your energetic flow.

EXERCISE 37: **Charging**

This is simply putting together what you have learned in Precharging for one smooth continual flow of energy.

1. From the zero point of Exercise 18, *The Clock*, inhale as you contract your PC muscle and bring your body to the twelve o'clock position.

2. This time feel your energy move up through your sacred chamber (second chakra), all the way to the base of your skull.

3. Exhale as you expand your PC muscle and bring your body back to the neutral position.

4. Feel your energy flow down your backside and return to your perineum.

5. This is one cycle. Continue for nine cycles or until your energetic track becomes warm and tingly.

6. Unlike Cycling which keeps you passively aroused, I find Charging to be more active. As such, I use it when I wish to instigate a hornier, heightened level of sexual arousal. As with Cycling, your movements when Charging will also become minimal as you primarily use your breath and consciousness for direction.

7. Try reversing the direction of your energetic flow.

EXERCISE 38: Dynamic Kegels

As opposed to simply performing static Kegels where all you do is tense and release, you have now learned how to incorporate both your breath and movement. The final step to making your Kegel workout truly dynamic, not to mention practical, is to be able to incorporate the postures so you can use them when masturbating or having intercourse with your partner.

1. When you have become comfortable with Exercise 29, *Cycling*, as well as Exercise 37, *Charging*, practice them in each of the sexual postures.

2. Once you can both *Cycle* and *Charge* in each of the postures, begin to practice them while you rotate through the postures as described in Exercise 14, *Connecting the Postures.*

   a. Focus on coordinating the rocking of your hips with a full exhale and inhale, as you contract or expand your perineum according to whether you are Cycling or Charging.

      • If the coordination is too difficult at first, then hold the contraction through all the postures while rocking and breathing fully. Next, do the same while maintaining the expansion. This is also helpful if you feel there is an imbalance in your ability to either contract or expand your perineum by giving you the opportunity to focus on one or the other.

3. Once you have learned to coordinate Cycling and Charging in each of the postures, use them while you masturbate and have sex with your partner.

   a. Note that Cycling is for stamina, as it will help you to avoid peaking and last longer. Used correctly, with a focus on the breath and slower movement, it will also de-armor you and your partner.

   b. Note that Charging is for power, as it will help you boost the level of both you and your partner's sexual energy. Be sure to pay close attention to your levels of arousal as Charging can easily cause either of you to peak. If you are approaching "the point of no return" switch to Cycling to begin drawing the energy up the spine before once again returning to Charging.

CHAPTER FIVE:

OPTIMAL SEX

BREAK THE ROUTINE:
THE RACE AND THE CHASE

Anyone with functional genitalia can perform the act of sex. Most people can get some sort of physical or temporary relief from it, though you'd be surprised by how many people do not. In fact, A large survey of almost 7,000 women in the U.K. found that experiencing pain during sex because of a condition called dyspareunia is incredibly common. The survey found that nearly one in ten women report experiencing painful sex, with women ages sixteen to twenty-four reporting an especially high incidence of painful sex. Painful sex isn't uncommon—according to statistics from the American College of Gynecologists and Obstetricians, seventy-five percent of women experience pain during sex at some point in their lifetimes.

Then there are a substantial number of women who report they're not deriving their own satisfaction from sex. Note that I write *their own*. According to Planned Parenthood statistics, as many as one in three women have trouble reaching orgasm when having sex. And as many as 80 percent of women have difficulty with orgasm from vaginal intercourse alone.

Most people approach sex as "chasing" 1) their own or 2) the other person's orgasm, as a means of achieving personal satisfaction. In the former case, this really boils down to self-masturbation, where the other person is simply yet another tool for scratching their sexual itch, "getting off," and getting it over. The latter is a masturbatory exchange *at best*, *if* the first one to orgasm is generous enough to return the favor, or *at worst*, the classic scenario of "masturbatory racing," where the first person to have a peak orgasm gets their cookie (normally the man), and the other gets their ego patted. The other person is then left unsatisfied to "finish the job" with their own hands or some battery operated/plug-in tool, or simply ignore their own needs. However, and not to paint too sweeping of a picture, these scenarios largely cover one-night stands or the all too common sexual plague of long-term relationships . . . routine sex.

For all hardcore romantics out there with some control over their clitoral orgasm and male ejaculation, sex may be better described as coordination where both people try to climax at the same time. The man paces his charging and the woman or man vigorously rubs away at her clitoris to experience the temporary, yet all too fleeting, high of a fifteen to forty-five second mutual peak orgasm. Either way, on some level, all scenarios are a form of "The Race and the Chase."

THE ROUTINE

Routines are static. They are also efficient, regardless of whether or not they are *effective*. They serve the purpose of saving us time and energy on performing, specific predetermined courses of action. Whether or not that course of action is fruitful towards our goal is something else, for routines are effective only when the given situation for which they were created is the present reality. The present reality, however, is dynamic, and unless working in a controlled environment it, rarely matches the specifics of a given situation. Instead, what most often happens when we succumb to habit is that we try to control the present reality so we can superimpose an effective routine. When this philosophy is applied to sex, the result is inevitably disastrous with a slow if not quick death of passion, excitement, and discovery. When breaking routines, it is not that we must throw out everything we know or do. If, on the other hand, what we think we know is fundamentally flawed, then we must uproot the foundation and everything built upon it. However, whether first becoming more cognizant of sexual choices or already being familiar with the practices in this book, the key desired outcome is the same: optimization. Be it a self-practice, single partner, or multiple partner practice, the practice must be interactive. For one's practice to be interactive, one must be expressive, so all participants are able to adapt, express, and adapt again until the interaction is complete.

THE IDEAL VS. THE OPTIMAL

An *ideal* is an abstract idea of same state usually based on what we imagine to be perfect, which in turn is most often based on some sort of familial, community, or societal consensus believed in by "everyone," but truly lived out by no one. It changes with the tide of hegemony, and can be as fickle as the advice found from one month to another in the latest fashion magazine.

On the other hand, the *optimal* is specific to a given environment and individual. The ideal is thought up, sought out, and validated through prescriptive application. The optimal is tested through experimentation, discovered interactively, lived out in action, and adaptive to the present. Idealists lean toward rigidity and almost inevitably become extremists when force becomes the only means for fitting reality to their ideal. Optimalists take the given tools and knowledge at hand and pursue the best solutions given their present state, environment, and company. Optimize, don't idealize, your sex life, and may your adventures be loving, joyful, and compassionate.

THE IMPERIAL SESSION

I believe, within every man and woman resides royalty, unique within themselves. Be it dormant or awakened, our bodies are temples of The Great Divine, and when we approach them as such we honor them. Sex becomes sacred, an act of service and an openness to receive service. The Imperial Session is the approach that has developed over the many sessions I have given to people and what I have been taught by their bodies' expressed and sometimes repressed desires. As opposed to taking this chapter as a prescriptive routine to dogmatically follow, I suggest using it as an interactive script for your improvisational exploration, otherwise it will simply become yet another routine. If anything, then it is an adaptive and evolving method I use to work with the body. Sus says that I should have my own name for it. So why not the Aaron Michael Method?

If I had approached the sessions I have given as a series of performed techniques, then the Imperial Session and Aaron Michael Method never would have developed, nor would they continue to evolve. There *are* preset roles to assume, primarily those of the giver and the receiver. The giver assumes the role of space holder, facilitator and guide for the receiver to express the release of any pain, discomfort or numbness they may encounter, and to open to whatever sensation, pleasure, or ecstasy they wish to explore. If you and a companion are taking turns swapping service, then I recommend that the Queen (the woman) works on the King (the man) first, unless she is clearly less energized. It will invigorate the man, get her out of her head, allow her to warm up, and relax her more for her session . . . which typically takes longer, and leaves both parties open and ready for sex to naturally proceed.

EXERCISE 39:

FOR HER MAJESTY: How to De-armor your Vagina into a Pleasure Palace for Squirting, Multiple, and Full Body Orgasms

On the World Wide Web, there seems to be a lot of confusion and conflicting information regarding how to excite feminine sexual pleasure and orgasmic potential, and there's a dearth of misinformation about anatomy. There are many questions such as, "How do I remove vaginal tightness, pain, discomfort, and numbness?" There are many more questions such as, "How do I have and maintain a pleasure-filled vagina?", "How do I regain sensation and bliss throughout my body, relationship, and sex life?", "How do I strengthen the pelvis and genital area of my body?", "How do I have an orgasm: clitoral, anal, squirting, cervical, womb, full body, oral, and heart orgasms?", "How do I create and harness my own sexual energy?", and "How do I allow, take, receive, give, pass on, conduct, jumpstart, or ground the sexual energy of another person?"

Orgasmic pleasure, as well as emotional or physical pain, exist on a spiraling staircase. Be it spiraling up and into pleasure or spiraling down and into pain, our challenges, rewards, fears, love and orgasmic bliss, come in cycles. Up the staircase, former challenges become smaller and resolve themselves more quickly while the rewards get more luxurious. Down the staircase, problems become bigger and take longer to process, while the benefits become more fleeting and less significant. Where going up the stairs may at first seem to be a harder, more strenuous exercise, in the long run it yields all the benefits and many more than what one may first feel when giving up and turning back down the staircase.

Did you know that with some simple touch, breathing, and voicing practice you can release pain from your vagina, as well as years of pent up stress, anxieties, fears, and traumas? Or that with a simple stone egg you can train, strengthen, and boost your orgasmic potential to supercharge your vagina with both the ability to receive and give legendary, bed shattering, earth-shaking pleasure?

This is written with the hope of shedding some light on the questions, challenges, practices, and hidden treasures women encounter along the path up their staircase towards ecstasy, self-discovery, encounters with others, and oneness. This is for all women who want to live fully orgasmic lives, free from emotional pain. It is also for those of us who love women, honor them, and wish to empower them—body, mind, and spirit.

To all the women who wish to come more in touch with their entire body and reclaim ownership over their sexuality, I am writing now specifically to you as I want to encourage you to find the time in your day to establish your own self-de-armoring practice. Not only will you develop a most intimate knowledge of your vulva's anatomical makeup, but you will learn to heal and relax her. There is no more powerful way to address whatever sexual healing for which you may be in need. You will learn the inner-workings of your pleasure, the distinct ways it can build, the different forms of orgasm to which it leads, so take your time. There is no better way to recover the erotic in your sex life and recondition yourself to be motivated and rewarded by bliss. Many women would be surprised that, as opposed to having to chase after ever longer, stronger vibrators, you can learn to touch inside yourself in such a way that when you breath, move, and voice your pleasure, your body will take over: your mind can shut off and orgasm can come naturally, continue as long as you like, and remain bubbling beneath the surface inside you as you go about your life. I recommend starting these exercises when your body is already curious or aroused. If you are desensitized or hypersensitive, then go without watching pornography, using your vibrator, or cumming on your clitoris for several days. When you do feel the arousal kindling then plan some time for yourself to either slip into a warm tub of water or cover yourself in coconut oil in front of the mirror. However it is that you go about it, do not start with your vulva directly nor try to go into an overtly horny space. Focus primarily on your breathing, voicing and movement as described in Exercises 26 and 27, *Genital Breathing* and *Genital Voicing*. When you feel ready, gradually approach your temple's outer chamber.

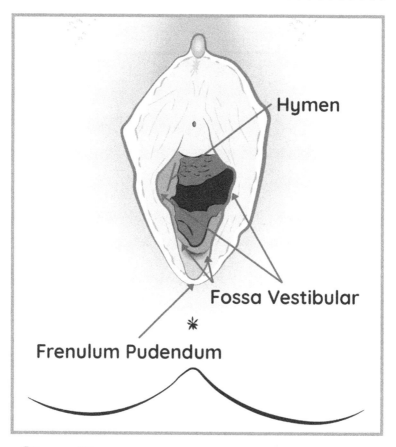

Diagram 23

1. With your finger, ever so lightly make contact to your vulva's frenulum pudendum and hold.

2. The sensation here can be localized to your vagina and, if storing tension, ranges from pain, to numbness, and releases into pleasure. Pain is often described as needles, burning, itching, acid or annoyance. Pleasure is often described as buzzing, pulsing,

swelling, and horniness. The finger giving the de-armoring to your vagina may feel releases of heat, weak to strong pulses, electricity, buzzing or burning coming from the vagina.

3. Continue to hold until the sensation in your vagina releases and melts from pain into pleasure. For the finger, this can feel similar to touching cold butter as it warms to room temperature, giving way to the slightest contact.

4. Gently dip your finger into the depth of the *fossa* (i.e. Latin for trench or ditch) just before reaching the remainder of your vagina's hymen. Hold as with the frenulum until your vagina's inner ridge begins to "melt."

5. Continue within the fossa and proceed 360 degrees around the *vestibulum* (i.e. Latin for the small room between the interior of the house and the street). With the pad of the finger, not the nail, gently nudge into the interior ridge of the fossa until it melts into the vaginal canal.

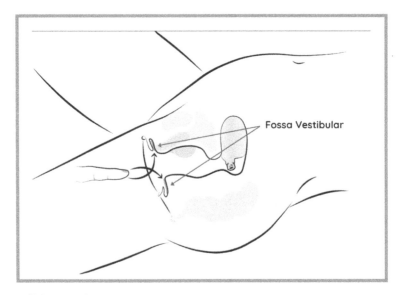

Fossa Vestibular

Diagram 24

6. If armor is encountered, then the range of sensation from pain, to numbness, and release into pleasure is similar to the frenulum, except wetter. As the Bartholin Glands are activated, they begin via the Bartholin ducts to saturate and flood the outer chamber with lubricant while the door to your vagina's inner chamber melts off its hinges.

"THE INNER CHAMBER" — PART 2

1. Lightly slide your finger in and along the anterior (upper) wall of the vagina. Your finger will come to a mound of flesh, here called the G-Pad to distinguish it from the G-Spot. The G-Pad, like any mound, has a slope on the front, as well as steeper slopes along the sides and back. By hooking your finger up and into the depth of the back slope, you will find the G-Spot which is more like a space that your finger can sink into and make contact to the pubic bone. Maintain contact with the G-Spot and gently along the pubic bone pull out and towards the entrance to coax the entire G-pad out.

(see next page)

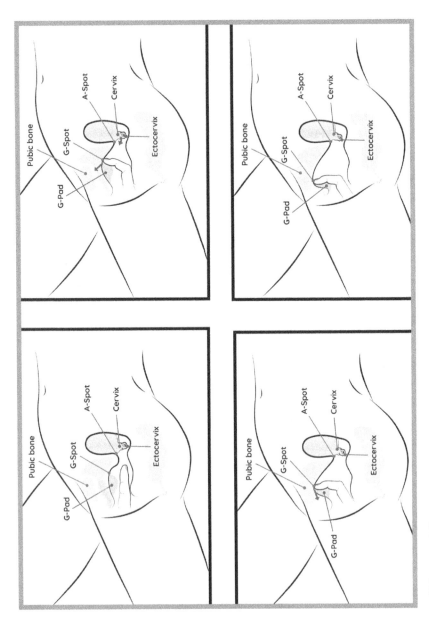

Diagram 25

2. The sensation here generally ranges from 1) numbness on the pad and pain in the G-Spot to 2) rip roaring pleasure on the G-pad coupled with the release of shame and guilt in the G-spot as you begin to venture with confidence into your true pleasure potential, unburdened from emotional pain. Pain is often felt on the side of the G-Pad more sharply than the outer chamber and can particularly feel like stabbing and needing to pee in the G-Spot. The finger giving the de-armoring typically feels releases of heat, strong pulses, electricity, and an overall fluffy swelling that snuggly squeezes the finger as the vagina releases into pleasure.

3. To counter any pain felt on the anterior (upper) wall of the vagina when pressing into the G-Pad and G-Spot, slowly but firmly pivot your fingers down into the front-end of the posterior (lower) vaginal wall at a depth of around one or two knuckles. This is also called the fourchette. Slowly stretch it backwards towards the entrance and into the Bartholin Glands.

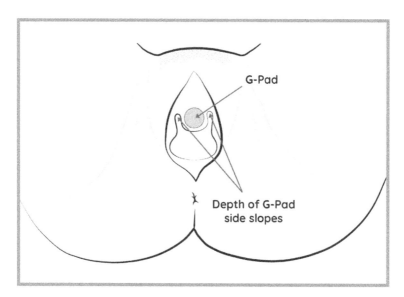

Diagram 26

4. The sensation as you press back into the posterior wall can range from a sharp, almost tearing pain at the frenulum pudendum (where the vaginal lips meet just above the anus and perineum) to a sensation of deep grounding and relaxation, which is most normally accompanied by sighs, deep moans and eyes rolling back into the head.

5. Remember to press and release all points of soreness and pain along the sidewall of the vagina. During the press and release, minimize friction and fast movements along the walls. If you have any sharp, shooting pains of electricity running down your leg, similar to bumping your funny bone at the arm's elbow, then this is a nerve and does not need to be pressed into.

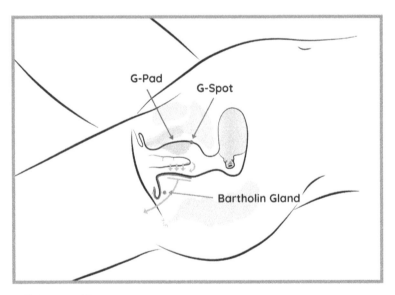

Diagram 27

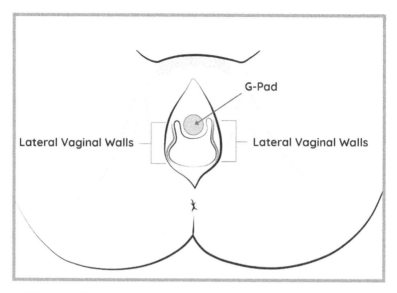

Diagram 28

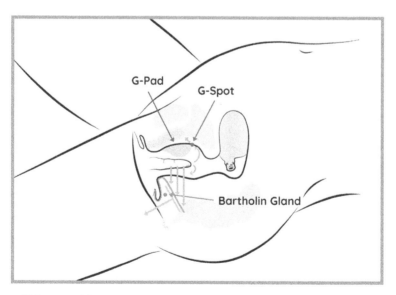

Diagram 29

6. Begin to alternate pressure back and forth between the Bartholin Gland using the back side of the finger and into the deepest point of the G-Spot, making contact with and then pulling along the pubic bone, with the padded side (not fingernail) of the finger.

7. Place the other hand on your heart.

8. Fill your lungs with air, arch your back, stretch your stomach and breath deep into your vagina, just like in Exercise 26, *Genital Breathing*. As your vagina's plasticity increases your entire G-pad will begin to come forward.

9. Voice without restraining whatever pain, shame, guilt, aggression, lust, or pleasure you feel.

10. Rock your hips backwards into the finger pressing into your G-Spot. Relax your hips forward as you exhale, the same as in Exercise 26, *Genital Breathing*.

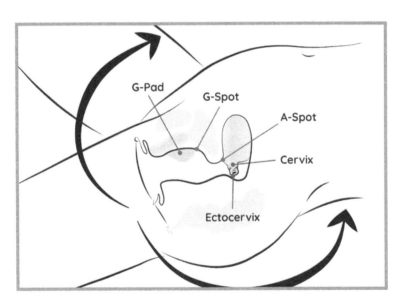

Diagram 30

11. Slowly, but gradually, increase the depth and rate by which you alternatively press into the G-Spot and fourchette (front-end of the posterior wall of the vagina). *(See also Diagram 27)*

12. To counter any pain felt on the anterior (upper) wall of the vagina when pressing into the G-Pad and G-Spot, slowly but firmly pivot your fingers down into the posterior (lower) vaginal wall and slowly stretch it backwards towards the entrance and into the Bartholin Glands.

13. As the rate of alternation increases to two to five up/down motions per second, the sharpness will begin to subside as the sensation of pleasure and a need to pee will increase. Go pee, and then drink a half liter of water.

14. Return and continue. Press firmly down and out, into the Bartholin glands and anterior wall of the vagina. The vestibular bulbs, like lungs, expand to maximum capacity as they surge

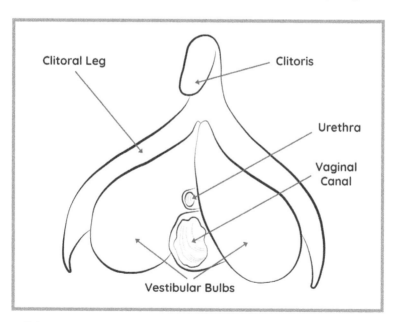

Diagram 31

full of blood, engorge your clitoris, and expand your entire vulva outwards while liquid waves of pleasure begin to squirt from your vagina when you press back up and into the G-spot, bringing the entire G-pad forward along the pubic bone.

15. The vulva fluffs making her lips pout. Unlike a face, a pouty pussy is a happy pussy!

"SQUIRTING: PHYSICAL BUILD-UP AND EMOTIONAL RELEASE" — PART 3A

1. Much more important than the theatrics of squirting is the physiological and psychological effects of female ejaculation. When first de-armoring the G-Pad, most women will begin to ooze a creamy, sometimes grainy, secretion. Typically, the milkier and grainer the secretion is, then the more build-up, pressure, and pain will be experienced just before release. Fortunately, even in extreme cases of sharp pain in the G-Spot and around the G-Pad, this pain almost immediately subsides with the first ejaculation and can be drastically reduced by, breathing fully, maintaining higher levels of hydration, regular de-armoring, and most importantly **voicing your root chakra tone forcefully** (this can sound and feel like unleashing a primordial roar).

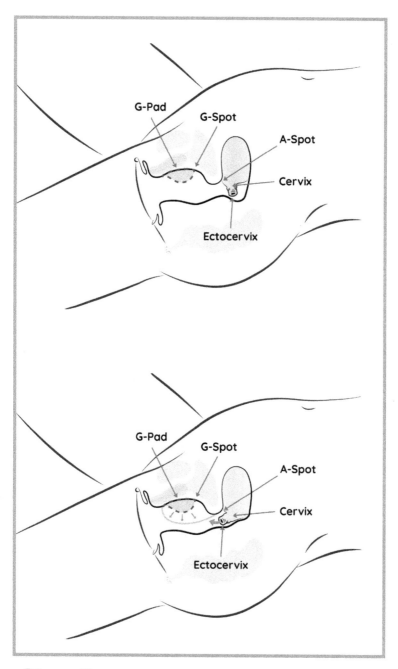

Diagram 32

2. In addition to the physical build-up, pressure, and pain experienced, these physical sensations are often complemented by the emotional experience of disgust, resistance, fear, stress, guilt, distrust, anger, shame, sadness, or anxiety. Eye contact, a hand on the heart, breathing deeply into the vagina and feet, and voicing what you are feeling, not so much with words, but with tonal sounds will create the most natural and powerful emotional release.

3. Go pee after the first psychosomatic release and then drink another half-liter of warm herbal tea or water (the benefit of warm herbal tea is that it will not lower your body temperature like cold water). The experience of peeing will also often feel like a psychosomatic release. The words most commonly used to describe the bodily sensations from this physical activity are "light" (in both its meanings: white light and weightlessness) and "cleansing." *(See also Diagram 23)*

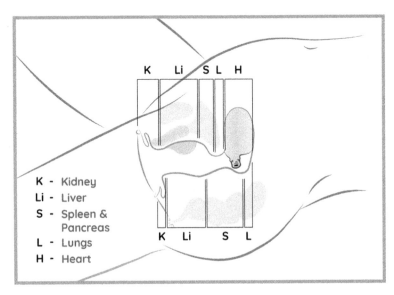

K - Kidney
Li - Liver
S - Spleen & Pancreas
L - Lungs
H - Heart

Diagram 33

4. Scan for any points of tension or rawness from friction or the up, down squirting motion. This can often times occur at the G-pad, frenulum pudendum, fossa vestibular (especially at the 6 o'clock on the posterior side), and fourchette (along the posterior side of the vagina). Release them if present not only with your touch, but **especially with your coordinated full breath, full voice, and full hip movement**. Stop if the skin feels raw. Return to squirting if there is still itchiness, burning, or more emotions to release, be they sadness, joy, or simply the desire to celebrate one's feminine abundance. Notice that with each release the ejaculate becomes less grainy, less milky, and clearer; the sensation less sharp and painful; the experience less anxious, angry, and guilt-ridden. Continue squirting and drink fluids until the ejaculate is completely clear. All negativity, like markings in the sand, is washed away by the powerful waves of new imprints. The sharpness around the G-Pad and G-Spot should nearly disappear and transform into gradually more and more intense sensations of pleasure and energetic pulsing. Ecstatic release, orgasmic potency, laughter, joy, soaring levels of confidence, a soft and juicy vagina, and a calm yet excitable state of absolute sexiness resides in the body and exudes from your voice, stance, and way of interacting. Some women, during the first three days, feel a bit vulnerable and lethargic if the negative emotional release was large. After all, ecstatic states and conducting orgasmic energy can be physically demanding as the mind (residing both in the body and brain) undergoes a systematic transformation in body language, breath, voice, brain activity, pulse, neurochemical and hormone production, interaction style, and focus. On the other hand, you may just go straight into maintained, heightened states of easily accessible arousal, as well as bubbling pleasure and horniness.

~~~~~~

1. In addition to the physical build-up and emotional release, the vagina literally transforms into an empowered state and anatomically realigns itself for deep orgasmic pleasure from intercourse.

2. The G-Pad and behind the cervix become engorged, tilting the ectocervix toward the entrance. The entire cervix and G-Pad reach forward so the size of the penis does not matter and allows it to easily reach the cervix, aligning its tip with the entrance to the ecstatic, dilating ectocervix.

3. Reaching behind the cervix into your vagina's posterior wall, fill up your lungs. Breathe deeply in your vagina, so that she reaches out towards the entrance and becomes shallow. Ever so lightly, lovingly and gently begin to pull the cervix forward. Hold all points that are sore as you work around the cervical base. Spiraling towards the ectocervix, de-armor the entire cervical shaft. Using a feather touch to begin, make laps with the pads of your finger around the ectocervix. Notice how the entire cervix begins to fluff and become soft. Remember that the cervix's reflexology corresponds to that of the heart *(See Diagram 33)*. As such, gently press the pad of your finger directly into the ectocervix and continue to deeply breath into your vagina and voice your heart chakra tone (see Exercise 25). Your cervix will begin to dilate as if to eat your finger. Breathe into your cervix so she reaches out like a mouth, at the ectocervix, opening and then closing as you relax through your outbreath.

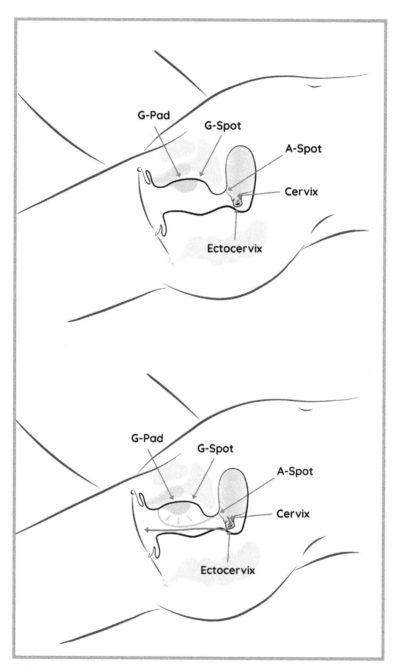

Diagram 34, before and after

4. Relax and breathe deeply. Hook with the finger pad back and into your inflated vagina's A-spot and pull forward along the pubic bone with the same motion you used with the G-Spot. When you now press into the A-spot, like with the G-Spot, your squirt, as opposed to coming in blasts, will stream more like a river.

5. Rock your hips backwards into your finger, stimulating the A-spot. Rolling your chest out, breath into your vagina filling her up with oxygen, love, and blood. The cervix will tilt forward, reach down, and push against the finger. Relaxing your hips, rock them forwards as your fingers lovingly brush backwards and tenderly press into the posterior wall of the vagina while voicing the root chakra tone in blasts of sound to relax the overall vaginal structure.

6. Pressing back and into the posterior wall of your vagina, gently brush the cervix as you pass by. Ever so gradually and lovingly rock your fingers backwards and into the posterior wall behind the base of the cervix, down and then gently towards the entrance, as with the G-Spot, but deeper.

7. Center the other hand on the heart, and with the center of the palm pulse in love.

The space-holder, facilitator, and/or giver should not taint the receiver's experience with words but instead simply facilitate the release. Where words may help, these behaviors seem to be foundational, favorable, and sufficient: observation, silence, and the eminence of LOVE . . . the latter being supreme.

EXERCISE 40:

FOR HIS MAJESTY: How to De-armor Your Cock For Take Charge, Rock Hard, Last as Long as You Like, Keep Her Fully Satisfied Sex

The roles for men and women in pop culture are strongly stigmatized with men depicted as needy dogs at a women's table of sex. If you, the man, behave and act accordingly, you will be gifted with the appropriate morsels to keep you faithful and in line.

In the long run, this exchange serves neither partner as "your woman" cannot, out of trust of you, "her man," surrender fully to her own pleasure, and likewise you will never step into your potential as the King invited into your Queen's sacred temple. The compliment to the needy male stigma is that your sexuality is considered simple where your cock is expected to rise to the occasion and perform when, where, and for as long as required. Though for some men this may be quite stimulating, you may find it overwhelming especially as you advance in years, your testosterone levels drop, or if you question the adequacy of your sexual prowess. By removing the tension, and especially the strict focus on sex, away from your genitals by spreading the sensation out towards the rest of your body, not only will you be able to cycle more sexual energy for harder erections and greater stamina, but most importantly you will begin to sense and feel into your lover's needs with your full body. Not only will you access your ability to unlock your Queen's pleasure gates to the most profound depths regardless of your penis size, but in turn when she accesses her higher levels of ecstatic bliss, you, her King, will be able to ride her orgasmic tidal forces into your own full-body, full-blown, and most satisfying orgasmic sexual joys (even without ejaculation).

YOUR IMPERIAL PENIS

1. With either your right or left hand, grasp the crown of your penis just under the head where it joins your shaft. Gently tug your cock out so that he stretches from the root.

2. With your other hand, wrap your middle finger and thumb around your penis's base where he meets your pubic bone and above the testicles. Begin to gently, yet firmly stretch the root of your penis by nudging and tucking it to the twelve, six, three, and nine o'clock positions.

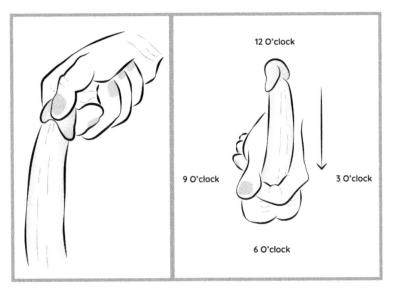

Diagram 35, from root to base (left); Diagram 36 (right)

a. Time your nudge and tuck with your voiced exhalation. Hold the stretch in place as you inhale so your breath, without the force of your hands, further extends your cock from your perineum.

3. Maintaining your grip around the head of the cock, place your middle finger of the other hand on one side of your cock's taint—the skin between your testicles and perineum—and your thumb on the other side.

4. Using the *Spacing* technique from Exercise 23, de-armor the base of your penis between your testicles and perineum by rocking it from side to side. Begin just under your testicles and slowly proceed all the way down your sphincter, working in time with your voiced breath. Your thumb and middle finger should almost meet on the backside of your penis's base as you relax into the applied spacing technique.

5. Maintaining your grip around the head of your penis, use your

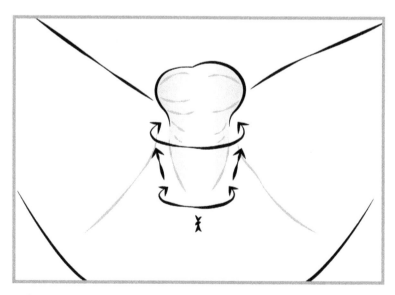

Diagram 37

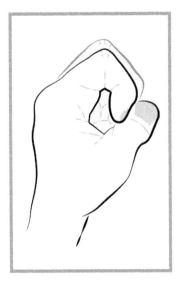

Diagram 38

other hand to make a loose fist. With the knuckles in the middle of your fingers begin gently to massage your butt muscles immediately around your perineum and anal sphincter by making small circles.

a. Use genital breathing and voicing to encourage your butt and anus to relax. As you approach your perineum and then your sphincter, breathe into your perineum so your sphincter reaches out towards your knuckles.

6. Reaching along your front side, make contact to your sphincter with the tip of your middle finger. Begin genital breathing so when you inhale your anal sphincter reaches out like a mouth to swallow your finger.

7. Do not push your finger, but instead continue to pull it in with your sphincter, as you breathe. Use Exercise 21, *Trigger Point Touch*, 360 degrees around the entrance to your anus, your first sphincter ring, and then the second. Be sure to breathe through and voice any pain, discomfort, numbness, sensation, or pleasure you may encounter as you continue to pull in your finger until it is fully inserted.

8. Feel along the anterior (front side . . . towards your belly-button side) of your anal canal for a mound of flesh anywhere from three to six centimeters (one to two inches) inside your anus. This is your prostate. When you reach the backside of the mound, feel for an indent. Gently hook your finger into your indent along the anterior (front-side) wall of your anal canal. Apply pressure towards and into your penis.

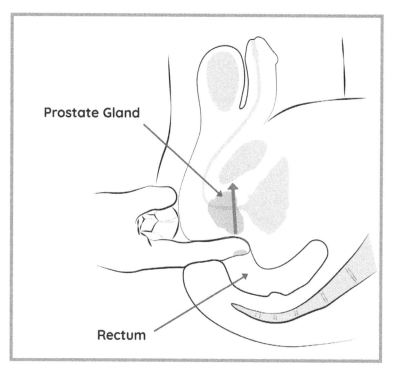

Prostate Gland

Rectum

Diagram 39

9. Begin genital breathing and voicing. Hold the pressure steady as you inhale. Feel your prostate swell onto your finger. Relax your prostate as you exhale. Gently and steadily sink your finger deeper into the indent with each exhalation as you feel your penis being pushed out and lengthened from the root.

    a. With each inhalation, as your prostate swells, the prostate should lower towards the entrance of your anus.

    b. The sensation here can be localized to your prostate, ranging from pain to numbness and releasing into pleasure. Similar to the vaginal G-Spot experience, pain is often described as needles, burning, itching, acid pressure, or annoyance. Pleasure is often described as buzzing, pulsing, swelling, and horniness, spreading from the prostate into the root of your penis and extending all the way into the tip of its crown.

10. Use Exercise 21, *Trigger Point Touch,* and Exercise 27, *Genital Voicing,* until the feeling in your prostate releases from pain and melts into pleasure. As the sensation shifts away from numbness, you may feel as if you might climax or that you have a need to pee. Pee if you need to do so.

    a. To counter any pain felt on the anterior wall (front-side) of the anal canal when pressing into the prostate, slowly but firmly pivot your finger (or fingers) down and into your posterior wall (backside) and stretch your anal canal backwards and towards your tail bone.

    b. Make contact with the tip of your finger, from inside your anus, to the tip of your coccyx. It is here where the sexual energy from your genitals will begin to cycle up your spine.

11. Apply pressure once again onto your prostate as described in step 8. Maintain the pressure while with the other hand using your middle finger to press into your perineum. With the finger you are using to press your perineum, begin to slide it up your urethra along the six o'clock position (underside) of your penis, while still maintaining pressure on your prostate with your other hand.

    a. When you pass your testicles, also apply pressure on the twelve o'clock side of your shaft with your thumb as you continue to slide up your urethra all the way to the tip of your penis's crown.

    b. Be sure to genital breathe and voice as you repeat step ten for three to nine times, or for as many breaths as desired until the tension is removed from along your urethral canal.

c. If you encounter any point of pain or discomfort, such as slight to sharp pin pricks or itchiness along your urethra, hold the point, breathing and voicing into the tension until the sensation subsides.

12. Remove the finger from your anus. Wash it or remove the glove if using one.

THE FAMILY JEWELS

〰〰〰〰〰〰〰〰〰〰〰〰〰〰〰〰〰〰〰

1. Make a ring between your thumb and index (or your middle finger if you prefer) and grasp around your testicles where they meet the base of your penis. As you inhale into your anus, perineum and balls, gently and gradually extend your balls down and away from your body. Repeat for three to nine breaths or until any tension you encounter is released.

a. You may experience anything from slight nausea, such as when driving over the top of a hill, or pain in the vas deferens or epididymis (the tube that connects the testicles to the body), to a sense of relaxation or depressurization in the urogenital areas. Be aware that, once skilled, this technique can be used to back away from the edge of ejaculation when approaching the point-of-no-return.

2. Release your ring grip from the base of your testicles and grasp one of them between your thumb, index, and middle finger. Massage your testicles by making nine, twenty-one, or twenty-seven small circles between your three fingers. When finished, do so in the opposite direction.

b. Repeat step 2 with your other testicle.

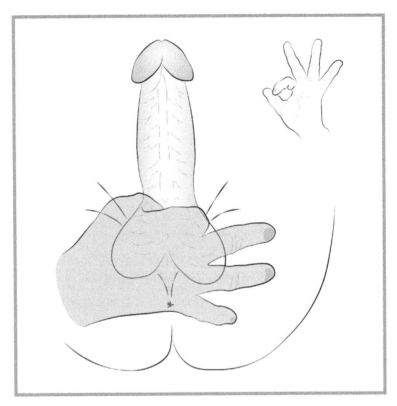

Diagram 40

THE SHAFT

1. Make a ring between your thumb and index finger, with the
   pinky side of your hand just above your pubic bone and testicles.
   (See also Diagram 36).
   a. Slowly increase the firmness of your grip so that your entire
      penis from the base through to its crown swells. This
      should not be to the point of pain but will likely be much

firmer than you expect a penis to be able to handle and such that the skin over your penis does not slide or your grip slip when you begin to pull out in the next step.

2. Voice your root chakra as you pull out in such a fashion that you feel a tug at the base of your penis.

3. Maintaining the pull at the base of your penis begin to slowly tug up towards your twelve o'clock for three to four breaths and repeat to your six, nine, and three o'clock. You can extend your tongue in the same direction, as its reflexology is connected to your penis and this will help you further stretch out your shaft from its root.

   a. Remember you should not feel pain, but again I emphasize that you may be surprised by how much pressure you can apply when gripping and pulling out.

4. Relax the ring grip. With your index finger, press into your urethra on your penis shaft's six o'clock, while applying pressure between the corpora cavernosa on your penis shaft's twelve o'clock.

   a. You will feel a slight indent between the two corpora cavernosa (The two chambers that run the length of the penis which are filled with spongy tissue.) With the tip of your finger pad (not the nail), wiggle laterally (from left to right) ever so slightly to create space and sink your finger in deeper.

5. Begin by applying pressure just above your testicles on the underside (six o'clock) of your penis, and as far under the pubic symphysis as possible on the topside (twelve o'clock) between the corpora cavernosa of your shaft.

   a. Following the urethral indent on your penis's underside, as well as the indent on the upper side between the corpora cavernosa, maintain the pressure as you slide your grip from the base all the way out to just under the crown of your penis.

6. If you encounter any small knots, which may feel like anything from dull discomfort or itchiness to small pinpoints of sharper pain, then hold pressure where they are and breathe into your penis. Voice what you feel until the sensation melts away. You can voice the tone of the organ from the Exercise 25, *Emotions and the Six Healing Sounds*, which corresponds to the reflexology point of Diagram 51 where you are experiencing the knot. If the sensation persists, take note of which organ the knot corresponds to as you may wish to practice inhaling and exhaling the appropriate positive and negative emotions.

7. With either lubricant or coconut oil, place the ring grip anew at the base of your penis and apply pressure. As you pull out, slide your grip from the base past the crown and tip. This should expand the crown as you pull out.

   a. As you reach the neck with your first hand, apply the ring grip with your other hand at the base of your penis. Release your first hand as you pass. Repeat step 7 with your second hand.

   b. Alternate hands, one after the other. Do so nine, eighteen, or thirty-six times until your penis feels stretched out from the base to tip, and on all sides like an inflated balloon.

1. Make contact at the bottom of your frenulum with your index finger as well as at the top with the other index finger.

2. Use Exercise 22's *Myofascial Release* technique to de-armor your frenulum. Some men will experience pain here similar to that of having your skin stretched, or in more extreme cases like tearing. You should not actually rip the skin, even though the frenulum may become sensitive or mildly chaff the first several times you practice this. Take it slow and feel into your body. Releasing tension here helps many men who struggle with premature ejaculation, be it upon initially entering your Queen's temple or later when unlocking her pleasure gates and Cycling elevated levels of sexual energy.

   a. Repeat steps 1 and 2 with one finger at the top of the frenulum and the other at the root of your penis at your perineum.

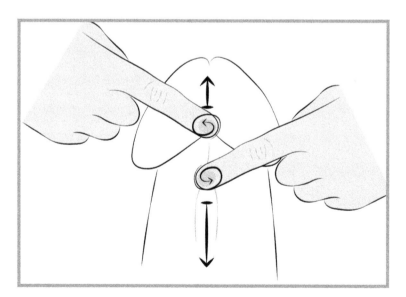

Diagram 41

This will further help to decentralize tension that can lead to premature ejaculation, by spreading sensation throughout your penis and connecting you to your entire self.

3. Using Exercise 21, *Trigger Point Touch,* with the pad of your fingertip touch into the depth of the groove where the neck of your penis joins the crown of your penis. Proceed 360 degrees around the crown. Even if your penis is erect or flaccid, the flesh will soften from rigid and bumpy, to smooth and fleshy, similar to the feel of a gummy bear.

4. If being de-armored by your partner, or if you're extremely flexible, then the tip of the tongue can be used as opposed to a finger. Moist, soft, without a nail, and able to be shaped, the tongue is an ideal tool for the job.

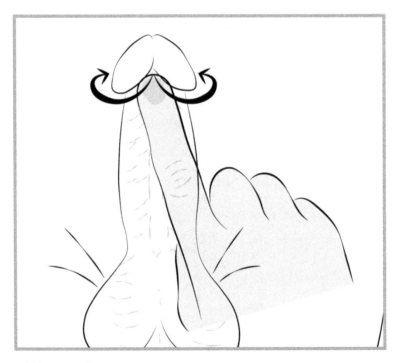

Diagram 42

THE CROWN

1. Grab the crown of your penis at the six o'clock (your frenulum) and twelve o'clock (topside of the penis head) between your index and thumb finger. Tilt your crown towards the six, twelve, three, and nine o'clock to stretch out the groove between the neck and head of your penis.

2. Inhale fully and tilt your crown to the six o'clock as you exhale fully, stretching out the groove between the neck and head of your penis.

    a. Repeat and use genital voicing and breathing until all pain, discomfort, or tightness gives way to a physical state of relaxation, and the flesh becomes supple to your touch.

    b. Repeat to your twelve, three, and nine o'clock.

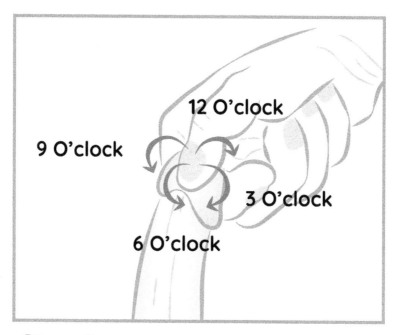

Diagram 43

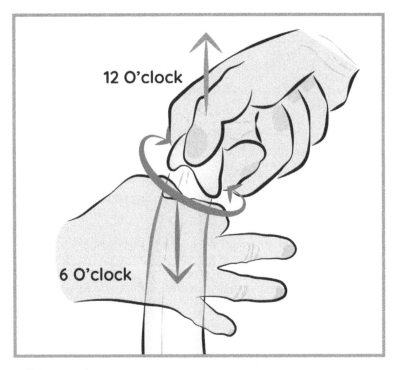

Diagram 44

3. With a ring grip, grab the neck of your penis, and with the other hand grasp the crown of your penis with your fingertips. Pull up on the crown to extend it away from the neck. Continue to hold the crown extended from the neck while doing your genital voicing and breathing.

  a. Inhale fully and extend the crown as you exhale fully. Relax your jaw, chest, legs, and tongue. Maintain the stretch.

4. Inhale fully and exhale fully as you pull up on the crown to extend it away from the neck.

  a. Relax your entire body as you exhale, especially your tongue, jaw, chest, and legs.

5. Continue to hold the crown extended from the neck as you inhale.

    a. Extend your tongue as you use your inhaled breath to stretch out the crown and entire urogenital zone.

    b. Repeat steps 4 and 5 while genital breathing and voicing until whatever tension or irritation you may encounter dissolves into relaxation and pleasure.

6. If being de-armored by your partner, then lips can be wrapped around the penis's crown to form a seal.

7. Your partner should slowly begin to pull on the crown of the penis with increased strength by gradually sucking more forcefully and increasing pressure within the mouth.

    a. The giver maintains the pressure from suction as long as they comfortably can by breathing as needed through their nose.

    b. Meanwhile you, the receiver, perform genital breathing and voicing through whatever tension or numbness you encounter until it transforms into sensation, pleasure, and ecstasy.

8. Proceed up the crown, repeating the same suction technique from step 7, one reflexology ring at a time.

    a. Finish with the lips wrapped around the urethral opening which can be quite intense for the receiver, who is voicing and breathing. The giver can place the Lao Gung point of one hand on the third-eye of the receiver. If dexterous, the giver can simultaneously place their other hand's Lao Gung point, while managing the cock with their lips, over the heart of the receiver to pulse in love.

MAKING MUSIC

You have learned the sounds of your instrument's notes and how to express them. You have learned some techniques for tuning into and tuning its strings. You have learned postures, movement, and how to give sessions for clearing away tension and emotional stress from your and your partner's temples. Now it is time to join together in the dance of life and make music.

EXERCISE 41: Connection Ritual

1. Face each other, both in *Horse on Knees* posture.

2. Each person should place their right hand on the heart of the other.

3. Next, each of you take your left hand and place it over your partner's right hand.

4. Look into each other's eyes and begin genital breathing and moving as described in Exercise 26, *Genital Breathing.*

5. Relax your jaws by allowing your tongues to become heavy. Maybe even slip in a kiss to help. Continue breathing and moving until you feel connected.

6. Inhale through your noses and open mouths, while continuing to match each other's breath with relaxed jaws. Inhale for a count of three as you gradually synchronize your movements and feel into the energy of your partner with your open palm and Lao Gung point over their heart. This is similar to Exercise 7, *Additional Tips for Identifying Resonance,* except that you are both inhaling at the same time.

7. Exhale through your noses and open mouths, voicing your heart chakras and directing your energy with voice and palm by focusing into each other's hearts. This is also similar to Exercise 7, *Additional Tips for Identifying Resonance,* except that you are both exhaling at the same time.

8. Maintain eye contact as you project compassion through your touch and eyes, allowing for all emotions to flow out, be transcended, and transformed into warmth and a tingling sensation.

9. Without breaking eye contact, or the contact of touch, use your left palms to caress down the left side of each other's body, over the hips, side of the butt, abdominal wall, and bring the hand to rest in between the legs so the left palm's Lao Gung point is over each other's root chakra as described in Exercise 27, Steps 1a and 1b of *Genital Voicing.*

   a. Mirror each other' s motion and breath. Take note of and feel into the other person with all your senses: smell, sound, taste, touch, and sight. Feel your body being touched as your heart energy flows through your partner's hands, connecting your heart's love, joy and patience into your root chakra. Feel the body of your partner, linking their heart chakra's love, joy, and patience to their root chakra through your hands.

   b. The energy will flow in through your right hand and into your heart as you inhale, and flow out your left hand, into their root, as you exhale.

   c. Be sure to remind each other, "Breath into your vagina/penis." You should feel your partner's penis/vagina swelling into the palm of your hand with each inhalation and relax on the exhalation.

d. Voice together your root chakras for at least nine breaths, but remain as long as you both like or until the root of your genitals are warm and tingling.

10. Without breaking the contact of your eyes or touch, the King takes his right palm and moves it to the right. Cupping under his partner's left breast and allowing his thumb to lightly graze over the Queen's nipple, his right hand proceeds around her shoulder before coming to rest on the Queen's wing point (Diagram 15: *The Micro Orbit and Energy Points*), between her shoulder blades and on the back side of her heart chakra.

11. Both continuing with *Genital Breathing,* the King waits for the Queen until she decides to release her hands from the man's heart and genitals.

12. Following her lead and without words, she will communicate whether to proceed according to 12a or 12b.

   a. The Queen moves into Posture #3, *Horse on Hands and Knees,* to open her throat and, therefore, vagina by fellating the King, while breathing deep into her vagina with each breath. The Queen can use one of her hands to guide his shaft into her throat and the other to maintain balance if need be. The reflexology of your throat is connected to your vagina and vice versa. Women, if in doubt, then cough with your fingers or the man's penis in your vagina and feel what happens. If you are more daring, then deep throat your man's penis and feel your vagina's reaction when you swallow or gag on it.

   • While you both voice your pleasure, the King begins to caress her entire body, softly and slowly, with the palms of his hands.

- Both breathe into your penis/vagina until you feel connected in your hearts and genitals.

- Once wet and aroused, the Queen guides the man onto his back into Posture #5, *Horse on Back*, and prepares to mount and take him in Posture #2, *Horse on Knees*.

  » As he is on his back, take him in with your eyes by exploring his entire body and watching his penis swell with his breathing. The King should watch her as she does so.

b. If the Queen has removed her hands and doesn't move into Posture #3, *Horse on Hands and Knees,* then the King slowly moves around behind her, so that both are still in the *Horse on Hands and Knees* position. His chest is now against her back. He places his right hand over her heart and left hand over her root so that his Lao Gung points are aligned with her chakras. With his chest against her backside, both begin to move in unison and to breathe into your respective penis and vagina, voicing your pleasure until you both feel connected in your hearts and genitals.

- The King guides the Queen into Posture #3, *Horse on Hands and Knees,* facing away from him. The woman breathes deeply into her vagina allowing her kundalini to dance as the man caresses her all over.

- The man guides her into Posture #4, *Horse on Side,* and then into Posture #5, *Horse on Back,* and prepares to enter her.

  » As she is on her back, take her in with your eyes by exploring her entire body and watching her vagina swell with her breathing. The Queen should watch him as he does so.

EXERCISE 42: **Entering Ritual**

Use this ritual as you first merge your bodies with physical penetration so as to ensure that no boundaries are crossed. Not only does this give the vagina ownership of whom or what enters her temple gates but allows the penis the pleasure of being fully accepted and invited to partake in the luxurious bounties of that which awaits to be unlocked.

1. Breathe into your genitals with the vaginal entrance a hands-length away from the penis. Line up the head of the penis so it is pointing towards the depths of the vagina. With each breath, the Queen's vagina should swell out and then pull in like a mouth on the exhalation, inviting in the penis to her cervix. As his perineum swells with his every breath, the King should try to feel from the base of his penis for the vagina's energetic pull.

2. Touch the vaginal entrance to the tip of the penis's head. The vagina should consume the head of the penis like a mouth, as both do genital breathing and expressively voice their desire.

   a. If continuing from Exercise 41, *Connecting Ritual,* Step 12a, then the Queen grabs the base of the King's penis and uses her vagina to pull it into her. When the head of the penis has begun to enter her outer chamber, she should angle it into her entrance's side wall and hold until any tension is released. When pressing into a point to release tension, the technique from Exercise *21, Trigger Point Touch,* should be used between the vagina and penis. The woman should breathe deeply into her vagina to push against the penis, and then exhale fully to relax her vagina and release the tension.

- Continue at the same depth, taking the penis 360°
around the entrance of your vagina, slowly feeling for
and releasing any points of tension you find.

- Take the penis in to the depth of your G-Spot and
repeat feeling into and releasing any points of
tension until you have gone around 360°.

- Do the same at the midpoint of your vagina, three-
quarters of the way in, all around the base and sides
of your cervix, and directly on the opening of the
ectocervix, releasing all tension, while you both
express your sensation with breath and voice. The
King should not hesitate to tell the Queen if she
needs to slow down because he is about to peak, or
a particular part of his penis needs to de-armor as
she takes him into her.

b. If continuing from Exercise 41, *Connecting Ritual,* step 12b,
where the King is taking the lead, then do the same as
Exercise 42 2a, except the King grabs the base of his penis
and directs the pressure where the Queen needs it at each
depth until contact with the cervix is established. The
Queen should not hesitate to tell the King if a spot needs
more attention and when he can proceed. Be sure that
both of you express your sensation with breath and voice.

DIFFERENT STROKES
FOR DIFFERENT FOLKS

The following strokes are just that, strokes. They are ways in which the male and female sexual organs can interact and stimulate one another for different effects. The positions I have chosen within which to describe these strokes should provide you and your partner the easiest means to explore the technique before switching around who is taking the more active or passive role. By in large, these strokes can be performed in any sexual position though the angles and orientations will vary, depending on whether partners are chest to chest or chest to back. In general, and especially when reaching higher states of pleasure, it would seem the woman's greatest challenge and blessing to herself and her partner is to open and let go completely to her dormant feminine power and pleasure.

The man's greatest challenge and pleasure is to remain present (not just in erection but in attentiveness), to praise, cycle, and absorb the explosive gifts and nearly insatiable forces of his partner's bounteous sexuality. As opposed to the gender-neutral term of horse, I use Mare to refer to Her Majesty's position, and Stallion for His Majesty's. Lastly, approach and relish each other as you would royalty, not in that you are confined to the rigid formality of court but instead with all the excitement and respect of a unique and powerful experience with one of God's most majestic creations, namely the access to one another's "Queendom and Kingdom."

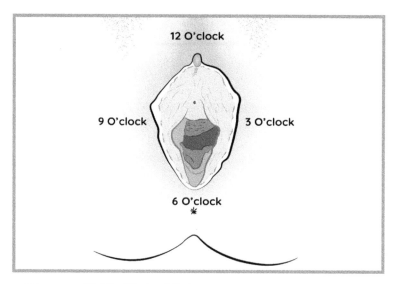

Diagram 45, The Vaginal Orientation

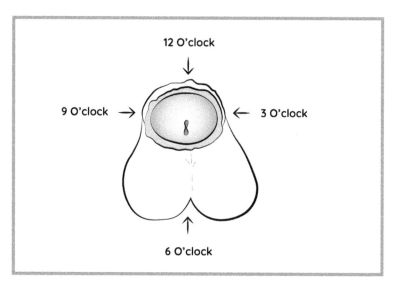

Diagram 46, The Cock Orientation

EXERCISE 43: **Come Hither**

~~~~~~

Here you will learn how to really stimulate the G-Pad with your joined movements. Ultimately it could be a penis, finger, dildo or other instrument.

1. From *Mare on Back* and *Stallion on Knees,* the King's penis is buried hilt deep and the Queen has linked her ectocervix to his tip.

2. The Queen is Charging such that her knees are rocking towards her chest while her hips are thrusting towards her twelve o'clock.

3. The King spreads his knees wide, to lower his body and is Cycling while he rocks his hips down and back to the 6 o'clock position. Alternatively, a pillow can be placed under the Queen's sacrum to raise the level of her hips.

    a. Their members are joined deeply. The effect of the Queen thrusting up her hips while the King rocks back before they both return to the neutral position is such that causes his penis to angle up while deep inside her. The top side of his penis works her anterior wall (twelve o'clock) from cervix to G-Spot as she thrusts up, while the entrance to her posterior wall (six o'clock) enjoys the bottom side of the base of his penis as he slides towards his six o'clock.

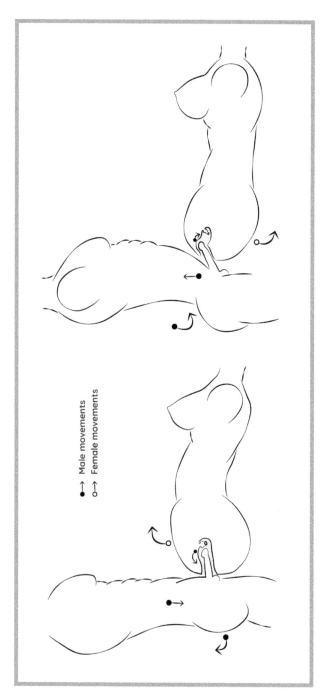

●→ Male movements
○→ Female movements

Diagram 47

b. This will prove particularly pleasurable for Her Majesty's A and G-Spots as the King's Penis will be performing a "come hither" motion. G and A-Spot orgasms are the Queen's gifts and bounty. Titillating his penis's head, the King will receive intense stimulation from the oven-like heat created by the rocking and pulsed contractions of Her Majesty's palatial vagina. His successful Cycling of the Queen's explosive energy can bring him to full-body orgasmic bliss.

c. This is a fiery and extremely horny stroke, requiring a well-de-armored vagina (especially around the G and A-spots) and penis (especially the topside of the head, when the partners are facing each other). Take care not to peak.

- Avoid reverting to simple in-and-out thrusting. Instead, use your expressive voice and deep genital breathing, timed with rocking movements that are more up and down than in-and-out, so you can remain connected as you gradually build up the sexual intensity.

- Due to the angle, the external portion of the clitoris will not be stimulated directly and should aid the Queen not to peak, while the King' s Cycling should help him not to peak as well.

d. The *Come-Hither* stroke is not limited to this position. The following are two alternative options.

With *Mare on Knees* mounting him in *Stallion on Back*, the Queen will be taking the more active role.

1. As both partner's chests are still facing each other, the hip movements remain the same for both parties.

2. By grabbing the King's shoulders, the Queen can add force, and speed to her forward-rocking motion.

3. Furthermore, by centering her vaginal opening more forward and towards his belly button, as opposed to directly over the base of his penis, the Queen will increase stimulation against her front wall and G-Spot while also lessening penetration if the King is in too deep.

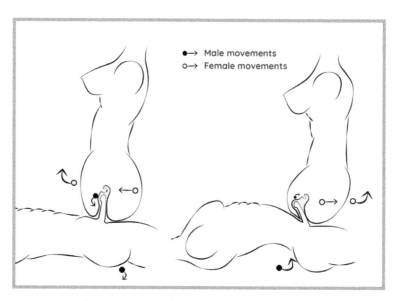

Diagram 47, Alternative 1

In *Mare on Hands and Knees* with him taking her from behind in either *Stallion on Knees* or standing in *Stallion Stance*:

1. The Queen is now facing away from the King. She will still charge, but he will now be Charging as well, not in and out, but remaining in deep and rocking up in the direction of her anus.

2. By grabbing the Queen's shoulders, the King can add force and speed to his forward-rocking motion. The King needs to be very connected and attentive to the Queen to ensure she is open for this and won't be hurt.

3. Furthermore, by centering the base of his penis higher and towards her anus, the King can increase the stimulation against her G-Spot and front wall. By standing up in *Stallion Stance* he can increase penetration if the Queen wants him deeper.

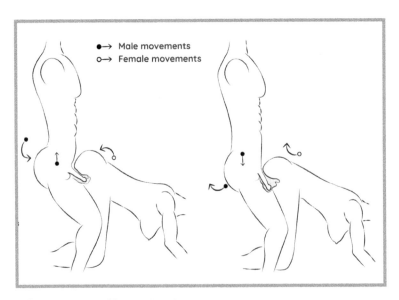

Diagram 47, Alternative 2

In *Mare on Side* and *Stallion on Side,* so the Queen is perpendicular to the King, as depicted, or so the Queen's back is against the King' s chest, the angles and positioning work the same as just described in Alternative 2, but is more intimate as the King can cuddle the Queen in his arms.

For additional effect, the King can voice and whisper how much he loves her in her ears while kissing her neck.

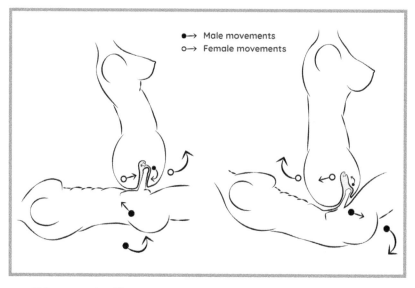

Diagram 47, Alternative 3

EXERCISE 44: **Take My Breath Away**

Here you will learn how to really stimulate and remove tension from the anal canal, fourchette area, posterior side of your vaginal canal, and out towards the vaginal entrance with your joined movements. Furthermore it can create a deep sense of relaxation and grounding as well as sinking into mutual trance like states during sex. Ultimately it could be a penis, finger, dildo, or other instrument.

1. From *Mare on Back* and *Stallion on Knees,* this stroke works best when the Queen's hips are free to swivel backwards. Use a pillow under the Queen's lower back to elevate her hips to give her a freer range of motion. Again, the man's penis is buried hilt deep and has linked the tip of his penis to her ectocervix.

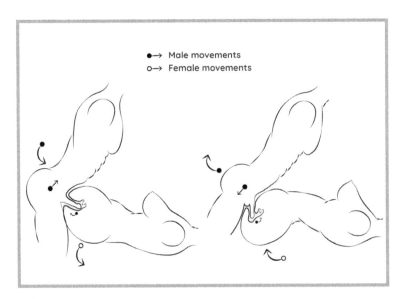

Diagram 48

2. The Queen is Cycling such that her chest, knees, and hips are rocking towards her six o'clock as she breathes *fully* into her vagina and arches her back. With her hips elevated by the pillow, she will have more room to rock backwards.

3. The King is Charging (not thrusting in and out but moving more up and down from his hips) towards his twelve o'clock with the base of his penis pressed firmly against the twelve o'clock of the Queen's Palace of Pleasure (her vagina) and G-Spot.

4. As she swivels back into his forward rocking, the Queen's pubic bone will press down on and stimulate the top side and base of the King's penis.

   a. This movement will cause the head of the King's penis to angle backwards towards her six o'clock, stimulating the depths of her vagina at the backside of her cervix and scooping back along her vagina's posterior wall. This stimulates both her back wall and anal canal, from behind the cervix to the area opposite her G-Spot as he rocks his hips forward and she rocks hers backward.

   b. The Queen's pubic bone will act as a vice on the King's penis, Charging his erection from base to tip, pumping it full of blood and rendering it into a steel rod.

   - As the King is on top, his erection will also benefit from the added effect of gravity.

   c. Expansive full-body orgasms can leave Her Majesty breathless as her pleasure balloons throughout her body while the experience of a maximally turgid, throbbing penis exploring the infiniteness of her divine feminine is the King's treasure trove.

   - This stroke is really opening and a myriad of emotions for both parties can surface, such as anything from cathartic tears to hysterical laughter of pure joy.

- Be sure that both parties breathe deeply and voice their emotions openly. With each stroke, breathe deeper and deeper into your genitals, allowing your voice and rhythmic movements to bond you as you freely express yourself in this dance of life and sexuality.

- Work together and be ready to hold space without judgment for whatever the other may feel.

  » If they cry, then smile lovingly into their eyes and continue to fuck (I use this word at the risk of sounding vulgar, for I wish to convey the forcefulness and intensity to which this movement can reach when both bodies are receptive and open) them wonderfully. If they ask for you to stop, then cradle them close in silence. However, do not try to "fix" anything. Simply be there for them. There will be time for talking and reflection later.

  » If they laugh, then do not become insecure or take offence. Instead, continue to fuck them wonderfully: join them in their joy, and pleasure them even more.

The *Take My Breath Away* stroke is not limited to this position. In fact, a skilled Queen will likely find *Mare on Knees,* riding the King in *Stallion on Back,* to be best as her hips are most free to swivel backwards.

1. As both partner's chests are still facing each other, the hip movements remain the same for both parties.

2. By grabbing the King's shoulders, the Queen can add force and speed to her backwards rocking.

3. Furthermore, by centering her vaginal opening more backwards and towards his balls as opposed to directly over the base of his penis, the Queen will increase stimulation in her anus through the added pressure on her posterior, vaginal wall, while also lessening penetration if the King is in too deep.

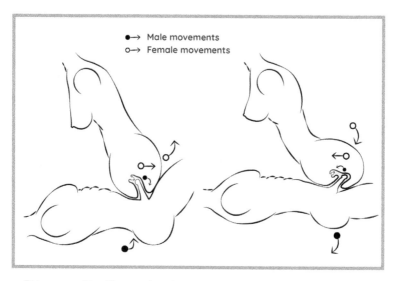

Diagram 48, Alternative 1

In *Mare on Hands and Knees* with him taking her from behind in *Stallion on Knees*:

1. The Queen is now facing away from the King. She will still *cycle* but he will now cycle as well, remaining in deep and rocking down and away from her anus.

2. By grabbing hold of and tossing up the Queen's hips as she cycles towards her six o'clock, the King can add force and speed to his downward rocking.

3. By centering the base of his penis lower and towards her clitoris the King can increase stimulation 1) on her clitoris, with the

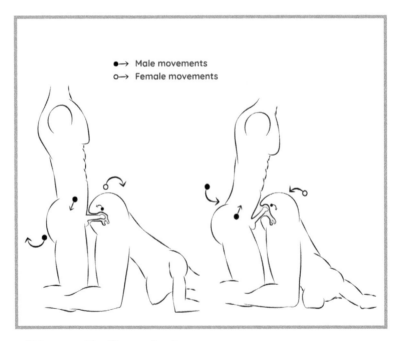

Diagram 48, Alternative 2

slapping of his balls 2) on her G-spot with the base of his penis, and 3) in her anus through the pressure of the head of his penis on her posterior vaginal wall. It will also lessen penetration if the King is in too deep.

TAKE MY BREATH AWAY – ALTERNATIVE 3

In *Mare on Side and Stallion on Side* so either 1) the Queen's back is facing the King's chest or 2) the Queen's body is perpendicular to the King's and forming a "T" relative to each other:

1. The angle and positioning of the penis and vagina work the same as described in the previous position, Alternative 2, *Mare on Hands* and *Knees with Stallion on Knees*.

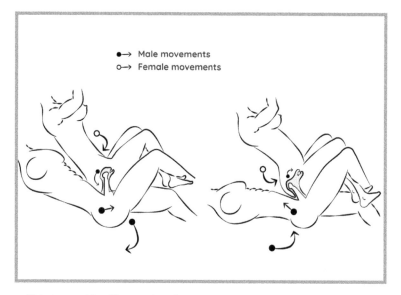

Diagram 48, Alternative 3

a. However, with the Queen's back against the King's chest the position is more intimate since the partners can cuddle with the King's arms wrapped around her back.

b. As the sex and horniness heat up, they can shift their bodies relative to each other to form a "T," so the Queen can swivel her hips backwards to increase the speed and force of the King's thrust as they desire.

2. Due to the angle, when the Queen is on top, her clitoris can become overstimulated by grinding into the base of the King's penis and pubic bone. However, since the Queen is Cycling when on top, she will likely not be clenching down, and the expansive breathing into her vagina will help her to avoid blocking off blood flow and overcharging her clitoris into a peak orgasm. Since it is the base of the King's penis against her G-Spot, instead of the head that is primarily being stimulated, he will be less likely to peak in spite of the fact that he is Charging. Lastly, when on top and positioning towards the King's balls, the Queen should be aware not to clench down or rock backwards with her palatial vagina beyond his capacity for pleasure. If his penis is already fully turgid, then it can cause him to peak. Worse yet, it can bend his penis to the point of experiencing pain or injury.

EXERCISE 45: **Exploding Hearts**

Here you will learn how to really stimulate the cervix with your joined movements, explore vulnerability, and connect your hearts. Ultimately it could be a penis, finger, dildo, or other instrument.

1. This stroke takes time but is well worth the reward. Before trying out this stroke, I recommend laughing, playing, having fun, enjoying other sexual strokes, and then trying it out some hours into the session. The Queen and her vagina should be highly aroused, *fully* expressive, completely de-armored (externally as well as internally along all vaginal walls), very open, and connected to her King (from her heart and cervix). Furthermore, the King's penis should be charged with energy, not having peaked for several days (fourteen or more, depending on the man

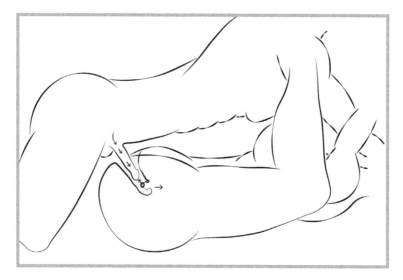

Diagram 49

and his age). Of course, you can enjoy this stroke sooner, but the fireworks will likely not be the same unless the King is especially skilled or, more importantly, the Queen's body is already primed through past experiences of cervical and womb orgasms.

2. The Queen and King align the opening to her ectocervix with that of his urethral opening.

3. Maintaining pressure on the point of contact, the Queen begins to breathe deeply into her vagina, lowering her cervix into or around his penis, depending on how dilated her cervix is.

4. The King should remain relatively still, focusing on breathing deeply into his genitals. He visualizes projecting his energy like a laser beam out the tip of his penis, up through her ectocervix and womb, and into her heart.

5. The Queen begins to pull her knees up to her chest and breathes through any remaining discomfort or tension in her vagina and around her cervix.

6. The King gently nuzzles further into the Queen's ectocervix. She will begin to dilate as her pleasure and openness increase.

7. On her inhalation as she cycles, her cervix should lower either into or, if considerably dilated, around the tip of the penis.

8. An energetic buzzing sensation between her cervix and his penis will begin. On the exhale as she cycles and pulls up with her PC muscles, her ectocervix, and entire vagina, like a mouth, will begin to suck at the King.

9. As the sexual arousal really starts to heighten, her cervix will become engorged with blood, soft and spongy around the surface, yet erect at the core. Insatiableness will overcome the Queen's vagina, and she will simply want to suck in the King further and further. At this point she can go into the yoga position, Happy Baby, for maximum penetration.

10. The King, without breaking contact, begins Charging energy as he pulses and taps his penis into her cervix with minute rhythmic thrusts. Through the Queen's erect cervix, vibrations from the King's Charging will cause her womb to quake with pleasure.

11. The Queen and King should gaze deep into one another's eyes and feel their hearts connect. Both should express themselves fully with voice, breath, and movement as the intensity of her Cycling and his Charging increases.

12. As the Queen's pleasure becomes hyperactive, she can let go of all inhibitions and follow her body's hunger. The man, responding to her call for more of him begins to increase the intensity of his Charging as he consciously nuzzles and pulses his sexual energy more firmly and profoundly into her dilated cervix. At this point the suction and wetness between her cervix and his penis can become so intense that the Queen's vagina can be heard sucking away on his shaft.

13. The Queen and King should press their chests together, and angle their bodies so their hearts align.

14. After what may be ten to twenty minutes or more of intense Charging, the vibrations in the Queen's womb will take on their own inertia as she begins to climax, sending waves of pleasure rippling throughout her body from her vaginal palace to her fingertips and finally exploding her heart into orgasmic bliss. Cervical, womb, heart, full-body orgasms and states of *satori* await the Queen who dares to open herself fully to her King in mind, body, and soul. Satori is a Japanese Buddhist term for awakening, comprehension, and understanding. In the Zen Buddhist tradition, *satori* refers to the experience of *kenshō*— seeing into one's true nature. *Satori* is commonly translated as enlightenment.

15. The double suction from her dripping vagina and hungry cervix offer the King the most intense pleasures. As he breathes into his genitals, voices his pleasure and opens his heart, her energy will bring him heart orgasms, sending him into full body bliss and altered states of consciousness.

    a. *Mare on Knees* mounted on *Stallion on Back* is a particularly good position for this stroke. This is especially true when the Queen is acquainted with the nature of her own cervical and womb orgasm. She will then be best capable to guide her King's penis into alignment with her cervix while she grinds into him just where it is needed.

    b. As this is an extremely energetic and demanding stroke, go slowly as you begin so that the Queen has more than enough time to open. Take your time throughout the build-up so the King can adjust to the increasingly powerful surges of energy from his Queen. To avoid peaking, the King can temper his Charging with Cycling as needed.

REFLEXOLOGY

As you become more adapt at the art of sexual healing not only will you use your hands with accuracy but your genitals as well, for they are truly potent and sacred instruments of empowerment. These strokes you have just learned focus stimulation on different reflexology regions of the vagina and penis. As such, it is worth a brief mention to note the organs they correspond to and the potential emotional effects that may arise if the organs are armored or out of balance.

1. Her Queen's G-Spot corresponds to the liver.

> **a.** When the G-Spot is armored, be aware that you, the Queen, may experience surges of anger and sexual greed. This may result in being uninterested in the King and demonstrated by:
>
> - Direct and outward verbal or physical aggression.
>
> - Introversion by becoming aloof, inexpressive, or unresponsive.
>
> - Repressed aggression by taking a disinterest in his pleasure or becoming overly egocentric in obtaining only your pleasure.
>
> **b.** Once the tension is released, emotions of gratitude, kindness and generosity will emerge as you begin to see your King's acts of lovemaking and the expression of your pleasures and female ejaculations as the gift they are.

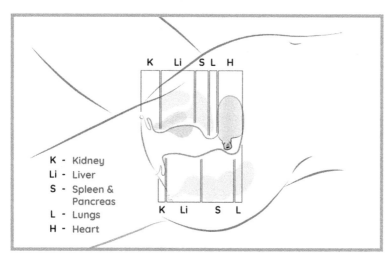

Diagram 50, Vaginal Reflexology

2. The area around Her Queen's A-spot corresponds to the lungs.

    a. When the area around the A-spot is armored, be aware that you may experience sadness and depression that can result in anything from tearing up to crying or even deep, heavy sobbing.

    b. Once the tension is released, feelings of sexual confidence and courage will emerge that will further overcome any shyness or apprehensions regarding sexual expression and female ejaculation.

3. Her Queen's cervix corresponds to her heart.

    a. When her cervix is armored be aware that if the King is too quick or forceful when making contact, she may experience intense rises in apathy and impatience.

- This will likely result in a (sometimes literal) knee-jerk reaction to kick him off. Sometimes the reaction is not as extreme, in which case the Queen may feel herself emotionally shutting down, distracted by "to-do lists," and wanting him to simply finish up.

- If the cervix is highly armored due to desensitization and the build-up of tension over time, then sex, as opposed to the joy it once was, will begin to feel like a routine for his pleasure, or worse yet, a chore.

    b. When your cervix is de-armored, slight or even intense stimulation will bring immense feelings of joy, love, and adoration.

- You will yearn to feel the King's body pressed up against your own. Internally and externally you will crave to have him closer and deeper. The feelings and pleasure can become almost insatiable and leave your body reverberating with pleasure and horniness for days.

PENILE REFLEXOLOGY

1. The head of the King's penis corresponds to the heart and lungs.

   a. The King should focus on breathing into and sensing his lungs and heart, expanding so as to remain connected and open to the Queen.

      - If the King's heart is closed, or the tip of his penis armored then his movements can be mechanical and disconnected from her needs as his apathy and impatience bring him to mentally zone out,

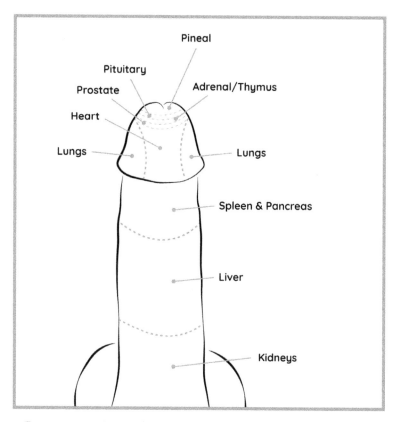

Diagram 51, Penile (Penis) Reflexology

focus on his own physical pleasure, or cause him to ejaculate prematurely.

» When the sex is finished, the King will likely want to roll away and be left alone.

- When the King's heart is open and the tip of his penis de-armored, he will desire and feel tuned into the Queen emotionally, energetically, and physically. He will wish to give and serve her with the act of sex, offering her pleasure and healing, sating her physical yearnings, and intuiting her energetic needs.

  » As opposed to wanting to be left alone after intercourse, the King will be cuddly, responsive, joyful, in love, and compassionate to not only the Queen's physical needs but those needs that are emotional and often surface post coitus.

- If the King's lungs are closed, or the tip of his penis armored, then the act of sex with the Queen can leave him feeling lonely, sad, and depressed.

  » The King may feel sexually used, unworthy, and doubt whether the Queen is truly satisfied, as well as feeling incapable of enjoying her or his own pleasures.

- When the King's lungs are open and the tip of his penis de-armored, then the act of sex with the Queen will leave him feeling courageous and self-confident.

  » During lovemaking, the King and his movements will be freer, explorative, and curious. As such, he will receive feedback directly from his Queen or intuitively from the interaction of each other's bodies.

CHAPTER SIX:

TOOLS

A GREAT PHOBIA AND
THE FINAL FRONTIER

We live in an age of information, where we have a multitude of reading material, pictures, videos and sounds accessible to us with only a few clicks of a button. Porn sites are some of the most visited on the World Wide Web, with pretty much any act, body part, and filmed angle readily available for free or pay. People watch all sorts of things, yet there are still a significant percentage of people who participate in the voyeurism of others, yet have never taken the time to inspect their own penis, vagina, or anus in the mirror. Even fewer have ever inserted their finger to explore what it is that they have.

A dear friend of mine had gone the first twenty-five years of her active sex life with men, women, vibrators, and dildos never having dared to look inside her own vagina—much less insert a finger. The mere thought of it made her physically sick to her stomach. She even feared she might do damage though, ironically, she would allow free-range to some guy she had met at a bar and only known for a few hours. Furthermore, she was vehemently opposed to inserting anything into her anus, declaring that it was "dirty," and "an exit not an entrance." Nevertheless, man-on-man action was her porn of choice for masturbation.

Sometime after we had raised the topic of her own fixation, yet aversion to anal stimulation, she decided to touch her sphincter with one of her small dildos. She later recounted to me that just from making contact to her anus's outer ring, she had become so horny that for the next several days she felt a continual sexual pulse around her sphincter. This in turn led her to masturbate multiple times a day and to rapidly climax on her clitoris with hardly any stimulation.

It would appear that there is a stigma when it comes to this form of self-exploration. Be it the discomfort of the unknown, or a great phobia of discovering hidden desires and likings when breeching these final frontiers, there are many therapeutic reasons to overcome these fears which have nothing to do with the pleasure of auto or other erotic stimulation (i.e. doing it to yourself versus receiving). The practices in this chapter will help you not only learn how to better cycle your sexual energy, but in many cases these practices can remove and cure years of built-up physical scarring or psychosomatic tension residing in the tissues and musculature. If, however, you do find enjoyment, then enjoy and do not get caught up on what others may or may not think. It's possible they feel the same as you.

THE BUTT FOR MEN AND WOMEN

Both men and women store a lot of fear, pain, and guilt around the anal sphincter. Tension here can cause us to walk with a stiff gait, as well as to adopt a rather inflexible demeanor and experience difficulties in relaxing. Men and women who find themselves continually peaking from little to no physical stimulation at all may likely be carrying tension in their anus. In these cases, I have found that it is typically the outer ring of the anus, as well as the prostate in men, that is tense and storing most of the physical and psychological pain, fear, anxiety, anger, and sorrow. On the other hand, it is the deeper inner rings of the anal canal that, when opened, create the greatest sensation of balance, relaxation, and being grounded. People describe the feeling as if the tubing of the canal were uncoiling as it stretched open. Not only does this facilitate defecation and alleviate constipation, but it makes us feel lighter with more internal space to better cycle our energy. Always start with a slow insertion, and you can douche your butt before beginning. If you don't have a douche, then just remove the tool, rinse, and use the toilet before reinsertion.

TOOL #1: THE PLUG

This is a great tool for working through phobias and taboos or simply becoming more accustomed to enjoying anal stimulation, as the plug can gradually be inserted and kept in for progressively longer periods of time as you do your daily tasks.

EXERCISE 46: **Intro to Using a Plug**

1. Begin *slowly* by simply making contact with the sphincter. Practice genital breathing so when you inhale, you feel as if your sphincter is operating like a mouth reaching out and opening so it can swallow the plug.

2. Do not push in the plug, but instead continue to pull it in until fully inserted.

3. Be generous with the lube. If you feel the plug is catching and no longer sliding in, then simply push it out and reapply more lube. Continue this process of pulling in, pushing out, reapplying lube, and then pulling it in again until it is fully inserted.

4. Once inserted, the plug should stay in on its own. From here you can practice genital breathing and voicing in the various sexual postures. If using the plug in the postures feels too sexual at first, then try walking around your house, doing some chores or even a yoga routine with it in to become more comfortable. This is particularly helpful for homophobic men or for women and men who associate the anus with feelings of dirtiness, guilt, or shame.

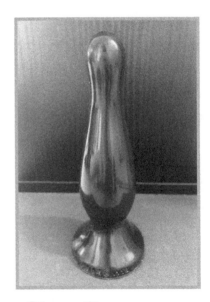

Diagram 52

TOOL #2: THE DILDO

These can come in all kinds of sizes and shapes and can be used to practice the different strokes mentioned for making music with your body during optimal sex.

EXERCISE 47: Intro to Using a Dildo

1. Insert the dildo the same way you did the plug. I recommend one with a suction-cup base, so you can stick it to the floor and slowly pull it in as you lower yourself onto it.

2. As you pass each ring, take note of any sensation of untwisting or churning sounds in your stomach.

3. Once fully inserted, practice breathing and voicing in a deep *Horse Stance* without moving up and down, but instead rocking your hips forward and backward. Just like Cycling, expand your perineum and anus into the dildo as you inhale. Pull up and contract as you exhale. You can increase the force and rate of your Cycling as your body becomes more comfortable and pain free.

4. Once you are free of pain and feeling relaxed, begin to

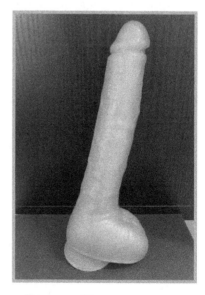

Diagram 53

move down with the inhalation and expansion and up with the exhalation and contraction.

5. The same way the vagina or penis uses Cycling breath, use this same technique to de-armor your anus. If you reverse the breathing process by Charging, then *you* can charge your anus with energy for anal orgasms and pleasure.

LE VAGINE: YOUR IMPERIAL GATE

My experience in the field of vaginal de-armoring and Imperial Sessions has made it obvious how little women know about their own sexual anatomy and capabilities. It is no great wonder, considering not just the lack of information but actual disinformation there is drifting about the World Wide Web regarding the female orgasm: how many or few one can have; what kinds and where; who can or can't have them; if it is normal to want an orgasm once a year, a month, a week, or all the time, etc.? The female orgasm (on the clitoral head) was only first scientifically recorded in the late 1950's. Even nowadays, many saleswomen sell sex products at vibrator parties (similarly to Tupperware parties) and discredit any orgasm that isn't clitoral as either "not really an orgasm" or the capability of only "the blessed select few" who just happen to be genetically gifted. To my knowledge there has not been any anatomical difference between the "two types" of women who can or can't have different orgasms (some researchers say that it is the distance between the clitoral head, vaginal entrance and G-pad but this changes as the your temple's plasticity increases and transforms into her saturated state). Well over ninety-five percent of all women who receive an Imperial Session with me ejaculate in the first session. Those who did not were those who chose to return and save ejaculation (i.e. confronting the initial emotions that can arise) for a follow-up session. In addition to the existent disinformation, the journey for women to arrive at their fully orgasmic potential is often not simply roses, chocolates, rainbows, and unicorns. As opposed to what is seen in the movies or described in romance novels, there are often a full spectrum of emotions and physical reactions, from sadness to joy, and laughter to anger, that you go through in this process of sexual self-discovery. The journey can slowly progress over months or occur in a moment. If both your partner and you, or you in your solo practice, give the needed permission, space, and time for all that may happen to happen out of compassion, understanding, and non-judgment, then it is not uncommon for you to go from exorcistic contortions and yelling to the utmost heights of ecstatic pleasures in one round of lovemaking.

It is the repeated experience of release, opening, and bliss where transformation manifests, healing occurs, and new adventures of trust, repair, and bonding begin between partners and within your own self. The most common occurrence women report after an Imperial Session is that they develop a completely different relationship to their vaginas. As opposed to a body part that you or someone else stimulates . . . *she,* your vagina, stimulates, invigorates, and informs you of your surroundings, the company you keep, and the decisions you make. No longer is your vagina simply your "baby maker" but it becomes *the birther* of immense joy, inspiration, passion, tremendous power, intuition, and wisdom. A constant guide, your vagina speaks into your inner state and health, while helping you to rejuvenate your outer state and navigate your relationship to, and gifts for, the world.

As with any relationship, you get out of it what you "put into it" . . . pun intended. Relationships are ever-changing, dynamic, and require time and attention. No two are alike, yet it is our relationships that breathe life into our living and put a hop, skip, and jump into our step. If you are well-acquainted with your vagina, you likely relate to her as a trusted friend. If you are not, then approach her as you would a new friend or a long-lost acquaintance who has just reentered your life anew.

Whether the relationship is trusted, new or reacquainted, leave room to rediscover her. Embrace her. Listen, explore and experience the world with her. From here, let go of "The Race and the Chase" and competing with other girls but instead embrace your fellow women as sisters, empowering them and being empowered by them. Cut out the "bad boys" who ignore, nag, and trick you. Invite and embrace the men who hold space, draw out, and celebrate the flowering of your divine feminine essence while unleashing your enraptured inner, sacred slut. This process of self-discovery and that of rediscovering others is, however, a *process*.

As you tune your instrument into a sweet music maker, your new resonance will attract those into your life who formerly would simply have been passersby on the path of life. Now, however, they take note of the vibratory resonance you trigger in them and their budding, sometimes inexplicable, desire to harmonize with you . . . be it just a gaze or much, much more.

An Imperial Session can be most helpful to place you and refocus you on the right path, yet it is not a substitute for your continued positive sexual practice. Here are some tools to further assist you in tuning your own instrument when self-de-armoring and nurturing perpetual pleasure.

TOOL #3: THE JADE EGG

Stine and our dinner guest had just arrived, when the internet cut out for the third time on Dr. Saida's Désilets and my zoom conversation. She was fascinatingly, lovingly and utterly re-educating me by dispelling many of the current day popularizations of the Taoist monks and nuns.

I got up from my work desk, turned to go greet our diner guest and then kiss Stine before excusing myself to to see if Saida was still online. A message over Facebook blings on the iphone "I'm not finished with you young man." I can't help but chuckle to myself as I picture the devious face she must have worn as she sent out that message with an ear-to-ear grin.

This was the popular myth I had read about across the internet and believed in until I had the good fortune or being set straight by Dr. Saida Désilets.

"The jade egg practice celebrates a long, cherished, yet somewhat occluded history. Beginning 2,000-3,000 years

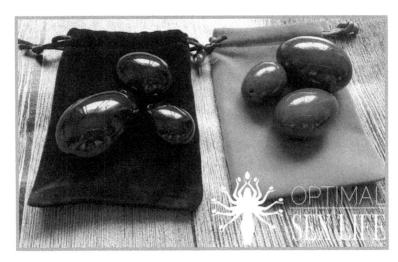

Diagram 53

ago, the practice was considered too powerful to give out to the common people. Endowing its practitioners with balanced hormones, longevity of life, regular menstrual cycles, rejuvenation, beauty into seniority, multiple orgasms, seductive prowess, calm, self-confidence, fortitude in time of need, and the ability to please any would-be courter with superior vaginal control beyond his wildest dreams, it is no wonder the jade egg practice was kept a guarded secret. Tibetan monks and Taoist medicinal practitioners passed on its teaching to the royal lineages, reserving the jade egg strictly for their queens, princesses and royal courtesans. The jade egg practice gave them an edge against potential female rivals, as those kingdoms possessing the knowledge were renowned for their sexual abilities and their hands would be sought out in marriage as a most precious rarity."

Nowadays, the jade egg practice has spread to the point of becoming a cornerstone tool for any female sex coach's arsenal of "revolutionize your sex life" and "teach your yoni the secrets of the cosmos" methods. However, Saida would be quick to point out that it is not the jade egg that teaches but your body that learns by using the jade egg. Dr. Saida was the first to write the book on the practice and is currently working with doctors and as well as other key people around the world to verify the magnificent results her clients get by daily practice over prolonged periods of time.

However on a global level, many people still are only acquainted with cheap knock-offs and Ben Wa balls, which are made of silicon surrounding a small piece of metal. Jingling while you walk, these balls cause the vagina walls to undergo micro contractions. In addition to being less sanitary, they lack the density, dimensions and the physical properties belonging to the jade egg for a wider variety of experiences and more complete practices.

Dr. Saida, told me that the accepted myth of the jade egg being a guarded secret of the Taoist healers, the royal lineages and their concubines may likely have some truth to it, but when speaking to Taoist scholars they have not found this in the historic documents. She did however say that whether made of jade, stones, or carved wood, there is a history of women for a long time that have used objects intravaginally in many cultures to explore and master the mysteries of their vagina with a likely focus on fertility. Saida even told me a story of a very powerful woman she met who lives in a cave and does her vaginal practice by sitting on a stalagmite.

As the modern founder of the jade egg movement, she knows that the interest most women have nowadays isn't to become an "Olympic Jade Egg" practitioner but simply to come more into touch with their bodies and to better enjoy their sex life. The results her students have are not just hearsay but have been endorsed medically and are currently being further researched for academic review. When a 70 year old woman with an early stage prolapse, who had never enjoyed sex, began a very basic jade egg practice with Saida, she went to have a pelvic exam. The results were as expected for a woman of her age and with her history of physical trauma. A year and a half later the doctor performed a 2nd pelvic exam. When the doctor looked at the results, awe set over her face. She said they were beholding a miracle. The vagina she had just examined was no longer that of the 70 year old women who walked in her door but instead that of a healthy 30 year-old. The vaginal wall of Saida's student had thickened without any hormones, and she was regularly experiencing multiple, full body ejaculatory orgasms.

Saida sees these sort of results consistently and with long-lasting effect, in her students, time and time again, regardless of age and background. More than likely if you are learning from someone other than Dr. Saida Désilets, then you are likely learning from someone who began their teaching journey after having attended a seminar of hers or read a portion of her book. If you ever have the good fortune to work with or even communicate with the beautiful Dr. Saida Désilets you could say that the proof of her practice is in the pudding. She embodies the jade egg practice, not just with a diploma on the wall, but with a lifetime of personal stories and experiences from which she can guide you. She vibrates with life, humor and vitality. She is fervent for maintaining the highest level of quality, professionalism and potency in the teachings she passes on to her students. In fact, currently as of Autumn 2019 there are only 12 practitioners in the world she has certified to teach her methods responsibly and to the highest standards.

I highly recommend working with Saida. In the same way, make sure the jade you use is the real deal. The effect of Nephrite Jade is especially good for grounding; balancing; as well as, both retaining and absorbing heat. With it, your body will learn to isolate each of *Your Priestess's* three layers to your pelvic floor** and truly master how to play her, as every woman can, like the magical instrument she is. Once you are in harmony with her hormonally, physically, mentally, and energetically, not only will you be able to have better orgasms and heightened states of pleasure in relaxation, but more importantly you will develop a two way communication to your sexual system where your yoni begins to speak to you. Your yoni will help you as you make decisions, communicate, think, and interpret the world. To find out more you may

---

** In actuality it isn't really layers either. Here is what Saida Désilets comments: "The pelvic floor isn't really layers, its more like interwoven muscles, so it's not like legos. I have found that I can train women (and myself, obviously!) to articulate the superficial 'opening' of the vagina layers with engaging the transverse-perineus and bulbocavernosus, then, the 2nd layer through engaging the inner most PC muscle/levator ani, and then, the 3rd layer with the iliococcygeusx/levator ani. and coccygeus/levator ani. At least, that's my current understanding!!"

o read Désilets's book, *Emergence of The Sensual Woman* ign up for her courses. She has generously provided a special offer to you, the reader:

https://vk250.isrefer.com/go/saidastore/optimalsexlife

In addition, Dr. Saida Désilets wants to break several myths:

1. In the beginning of the jade egg practice you may not even use the egg. In fact, she recommends using your own finger to connect and begin to feel the pulse of your vagina.

2. You do not push in the egg but instead it is your yoni that opens like a mouth, invites in and swallows the egg. Saida actually recommends yawning with your mouth to open your throat. Due to the reflexological relation between the throat and vagina, yawning with one mouth helps to yawn open the other.

3. It is not by contracting the pelvic floor muscles that you keep in the egg but instead by healthy, toned, supple and dexterous musculature. When done correctly, it is not an issue to keep an egg in for an entire day.

4. The practice is cumulative, and it is better to do 5 minutes a day as opposed to an hour once a month.

Her stringing and cleaning exercises are on the following pages, and can also be found at the link below if you would like access to them online:

https://vk250.isrefer.com/go/jadeegg/optimalsexlife

EXERCISE 48: **Cleaning and Stringing**

Following is an exercise for the initial cleaning and stringing of your stone egg:

1. Take your jade or obsidian yoni eggs out of the pouch and place them in a pot with lukewarm water. It is important that the water is not already boiling (an added precaution to prevent your egg from cracking due to a rapid temperature change).

2. Turn on the heat until the water beings to boil. Let them boil for 60 seconds before removing the pot from the heat.

3. Allow the egg to cool for approximately 20 minutes on its own, then remove it from the water.

4. Ensure that there is no calcium build up on the surface of the egg due to boiling them in the water.

    a. If your egg no longer looks smooth nor has its natural polish, just buff it with a cotton cloth.

5. Give your egg a rinse in water that you find to be a desirable temperature. You can touch the egg to your inner thigh or nose before inserting it, in order to test if it will be too hot or cold for your liking.

6. Measure out a length of non-bleached, wax-free dental floss so that when you double it, it runs approximately the length of your elbow to the tip of your middle finger.

7. Insert the doubled string through the eye of the jade egg, and make a lark's head knot by looping the string's two loose ends back through where the string is doubled.

8. Bring your egg close enough to your pussy's entrance so that when you begin to breathe and voice, as described in Exercises

26 and 27, *Genital Breathing* and *Genital Voicing*, your sexual temple can reach out and make contact to your egg.

9. Take time to feel into whether or not your body, and specifically the sensations around your pussy, are telling you that she wants to bring the egg in further.

   a. If not, then take away the egg and return to try again at a later time.

   b. If yes, then gently push out your pussy as you inhale and pull in the egg by contracting your pussy to suck up the egg like a mouth when you exhale and voice your root chakra.

Follow the link below to find Dr. Saida Désilets' medically endorsed jade egg course, future courses, or to purchase your own 100% authentic nephrite jade egg while supplies last:

https://vk250.isrefer.com/go/saidastore/optimalsexlife

TOOL #4: THE JADE SHAKTI STICK

These are majestic tools and forces of nature as they combine the best of a dildo and the earthly properties of stone eggs into one. The Shakti stick is a powerful tool and can quickly become your favorite play toy as well. You can use it in the same way you would your fingers, as described in Exercises 21-23 under the section De-armoring and Exercise 39, *The Imperial Session for Her Majesty*. For insertion you can refer to Exercise 42, *Entering Ritual*. Where the angles can be difficult to use your finger, the Shakti stick gives you greater access to your vagina and especially your cervix. It is an excellent tool for self-de-armoring as well as accessing your deeper levels of pleasure and orgasm by guiding it like a penis in Exercises 43-45. Furthermore, refer to the cleaning, insertion and meditative exercises of the jade egg practices.

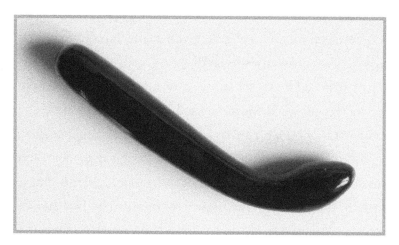

Diagram 55

LE COCK

My time at military school, sports camp, and in general at all-male gatherings has showed me that where women know little about their own sexual capabilities, men presume that they know everything they need to know. Listening, one would think this knowledge was somehow born into us through our genetic makeup. With women, knowing little leads to curiosity. Whereas with men "knowing everything" leads to ignorance, seasoned with arrogance. Furthermore, the oftentimes endless jokes about who is gay, the posturing to establish dominance, and the braggart storytelling about their penises as swords for conquering and gaining advantage over others would, in my opinion, lead anyone with an objective mind to the conclusion that the vast majority of men were either latent homosexual rapists, sugar-coated in homophobia, or simply contentedly ignorant persons insecure in their masculinity.

However, we men are gifted with so much more than that for which we give ourselves credit.

As opposed to sword swingers, we can be key masters to the secrets of the feminine sacred chamber. As opposed to simple warriors, we can be shamans. We are supposed to be the medicine men and musicians designed to heal and fine-tune the magnificent musical instrument and gift that is woman. If we had half the respect for our own bodies, and an accurate knowledge of what we are truly capable of, then a socio-sexual revolution would be eminent.

Our sisters are awakening to the fact that they have wanted and deserved more out of their sexuality than has been allotted to them in recent history. They are embracing and reclaiming their sexual power and desires. If men simply stepped into the roles for which we are desired, and as such assumed responsibility for the gift our penises are, then the paradigm of men having to chase, trick, trade, persuade, or buy women into bed would be turned on its head. As opposed to getting hard-ons from our own needy lust, our penises, like a compass, would respond to the magnetic pull of our women's internal universes. Capable of setting their cosmos in motion, we would find them open, willing, and desiring the light and heat of our fire. Their call to make the sweet music of love, adoration, and praise to the All would have us swimming in female abundance and satisfaction far beyond any locker-room braggart's ramblings. So, men, open your minds and train your penises, so they may serve you and those in your intimate life. In this vein, here is a powerful tool to aid you in your quest towards the optimal sex life.

TOOL #5: SOUNDS

Though not made of stainless steel, the Romans used tools such as these. Van Buren Sounds are extremely powerful tools for de-armoring the penis and maintaining penile health. Here I have included an exercise, like many of those found in this book, that you will likely find nowhere else. Bravery is

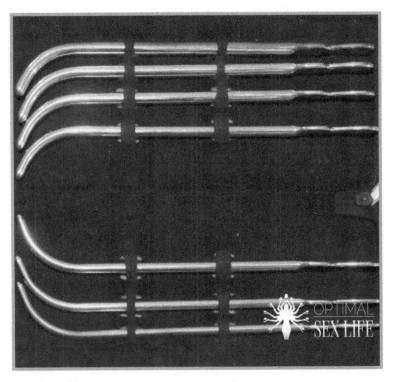

Diagram 56: Picture of Van Buren sounds

rewarded for those who wish to unlock hidden powers, literally from within their own cock.

As I mentioned in previous chapters, something had cut my penis from the inside. After about five years, my penis had partially healed, but it was still only working at sixty to seventy percent capacity at best. I could feel something was still lodged where my urethra joined my bladder. Before my injury, when pre-semen would begin to seep out, I would feel no discomfort and continue reaching higher and higher levels of energetic sex; giving deeper and deeper levels of profoundly curative and sating satisfaction to my partner. However, post-injury, the pre-semen would trigger an internal irritation and burning sensation right where I felt something was lodged, as well as a swelling on my penis's head at my urethral opening.

I spoke to several doctors and urologists about this condition but in general they didn't listen. It wasn't until I spoke to a doctor in Denmark that the option was first even mentioned of using a camera to look inside. After this and for whatever reason—possibly wishful thinking on my part—the irritation seemed to subside during erection and I thought the situation had taken care of itself. Maybe it was the buildup of distrust in the medical community at large by this point, but I decided not to go for the inspection.

Not long after this, however, I noted that the issue persisted, and I still felt limited in my sexual potential. Nearly nine years had passed since the fateful day of my injury, yet at the first neotantra workshop my wife and I attended, I felt led to speak with one of the bodyworkers about it. He mentioned to me a tool he had never used personally but had heard about, and that I might find helpful. *Sounds,* he told me, were metal tools I could insert through my urethral opening and down into my penis to de-armor it from within. After the workshop, I visited our city's local sex shop and found a diverse display of various assorted metal tools and sex toys. There was one straight, small metal piece about five centimeters (about two inches) in length as well as a large eight-piece set of Van Buren sounds, more commonly known as J-sounds. The Van Buren sounds were long, and the set was expensive, ranging in girth with a numbering system ranging from 18 for the thinnest and 32 for the thickest. As I was only currently feeling pain in my shaft, I thought I only had to remove some scar tissue. So, I bought the single, smaller sound and began to use it in my daily practice. Applying coconut oil, I began rubbing into and stretching out where I could feel some scar tissue had accumulated. Yet once the scar tissue had been removed, I once again began to feel that something was still lodged. The de-armoring with the small piece had re-sensitized me, and I could feel then, more than I had in a long time, that there was still an obstruction.

When the Van Buren set would not leave my mind, I went directly to the store, bought it, and immediately put it to use. I began with 18Fr, which is the French catheter scale and translates into 6 mm in diameter. It was pleasurable and there was a little bleeding when I pissed. I then proceeded to 20Fr. There, more pleasure and a little more bleeding. Finally, at 22Fr, the piece held firm where the urethra and the bladder connect. I chanted a long low *uuuuuuuuh* deep into my root chakra and the sound (pun intended) sunk in. With the J-hooked sound, I worked the bladder walls, especially around the entrance where there were some sharp points of pain. The sharpness turned to a mild itchiness and headed towards some sort of pleasure. This time, when I went to piss the stream did not come easy and was accompanied with a ring of tension registering like pain, where my urethra connects to my bladder. As the pressure of the stream built, so did the tension. I don't know how else to describe it, but the tension broke and felt like what I imagine to be the breaking of a hymen. Something black with coagulated blood around it shot out, hit the side of the toilet bowl and stuck as my stream opened, unhindered. An intense electric current began to stream through where the tension broke. It felt like burning, microscopic, electric needles were stitching together my penis from the inside out, from where the bladder met the urethra to the tip of my penis. My penis got hot and turned a darker hue of red and purple. Though not turgid, it began to point straight out, and a strong buzzing from within began. I was filled with pain, pleasure, and praise as I thanked God. I returned to the sounds: 24Fr (pleasure and ease); 26Fr (more pleasure and ease); 28Fr (more and more); 30Fr (slides in easy). At 32Fr, the largest in the set and a piece which stood out in my mind, the insertion was slower than the rest. Twice I had to relax deeper before it passed into my bladder. Relaxing my penis to allow the sound to enter reminded me of the times I had seen women relax their vaginas as I penetrated them. So, like a vagina can do with a penis, I discovered I could pull in or push out the sound with my penis. The buzzing in my penis intensified. When I removed the sound, the hue darkened further. My penis, though limp, pointed out straight and an intense buzzing, like that of a tuning fork freshly struck, about two to three centimeters (roughly three-quarters of an inch to a bit over an inch) out past the tip of my cock set in.

I bicycled to my Danish class, which consisted mainly of females, and ran into mostly women along the way. Just trying to navigate the crazy amount of sensation I was feeling, in combination with the loads of fluid I had drank and the subsequent need to piss, made me less inclined to be social. Nevertheless, women continued to engage me in conversation, with eye contact, and wide, flashing teeth-out smiles (not a common site to behold on the faces of Scandinavian female strangers, which more often than not carry a sterner, more masculine front).

That night and the following morning, my wife and I fucked (again I use this word at the risk of offense but to express the intensity of the energy and motion we exercised) each other's brains out. My cock was charged and powerful. Fucking her deep and working her cervix I felt both ridiculously masculine, yet fully in touch with my feminine as her cervix nuzzled into the entrance of my penis tip. Energy streams and muscle memories from before the injury eight years prior came flooding back. No longer was I regulating pleasure levels but feeling into and expanding their limits. Since the breaking of my "man-hymen" I have been filled with an abundance of gratitude, heightened energy coursing through my penis, and a desire to serve—the female tribe and their partners.

Since then, I have passed on this practice to many men. They too noticed a greater ability to circulate higher levels of sexual energy, a most thoroughly de-armored penis, a better understanding and empathy towards how a woman feels when penetrated, a greater understanding of how to penetrate her, and a more precise ability to *Cycle* and *Charge,* especially when joining their penis tip to interact with the Queen's cervix. The benefits for those men who overcome their initial terrors of pain will find their fears vapid, and the benefits for them and their partner ample. Be brave and enjoy taking your penis's abilities to the next level.

The following are exercises for the initial cleaning, insertion and de-armoring with a Van Buren sound.

EXERCISE 48: **How to Clean**

1. Take your sound set pieces and place them in boiling water.
2. Let them boil for at least 60 seconds before removing the pot from the heat.
3. Ensure that there is no calcium build up on the surface of the sound set pieces from boiling them in the water.
   a. If the sound set pieces no longer look smooth or any have lost their natural polish, then buff with a cotton cloth.

EXERCISE 49: **What You Will Need to Get Started**

1. One cock . . . wash him entirely and especially around the head before starting.
2. Two to three liters of water, cold or hot
   a. Cold water will drop your temperature and make your cock shorter and stiffer, but less likely to get erect.
   b. Warm water, such as tea, will make the cock softer but longer. There is not a big chance you will get erect when you first navigate the psychology of inserting metal rods into your cock.
3. Organic coconut oil
4. You can find Van Buren sound sets that come in sizes 18-32.
   a. Do not go smaller than 18 if you are a beginner. In general, the thicker the piece you can fit, the safer it is for you.

EXERCISE 50: **External Coordination and Insertion**

1. From a standing or sitting position, you are looking down.

2. Hold your cock's tip up to your belly button.

   a. Your cock's tip will be at the North.

   b. Down between your knees is South.

   c. To your left is East, and to your right is West.

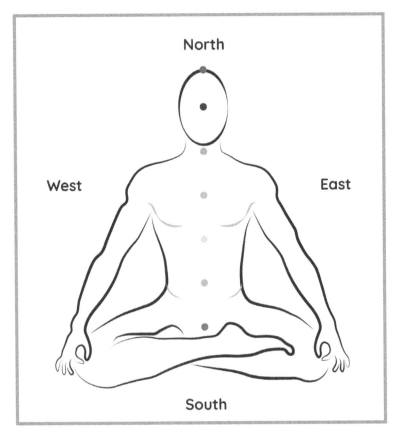

Diagram 57

3. Motion along the line running perpendicular to your body, we will call movement along the zero point.

4. Continue to hold your cock up and go over to a mirror. Position yourself for a side profile view with your shoulder facing the mirror. Note the shape of your cock as he goes down beneath your testicles and then hooks back up and into your body. It is like the capital letter "J," which is the same shape as the Van Buren sound.

a. The base of the letter would be your perineum.

b. Your urethral tube follows this path back into the bladder's opening.

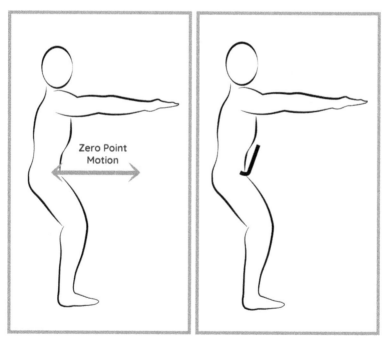

Diagram 58   *Diagram 59*

5. With your cock at the North, hook the sound in like you would bait a shrimp. *(Diagram 60)*

   a. I recommend sitting on the edge of the bed for the first time . . . facing a mirror.

   b. Think pussy . . . think of how you would tell a woman to breath and voice her root chakra (say *uhhhhhh*) as she welcomed in your key to her temple gates.

   c. Do not push the sound in . . . Instead allow the coconut oil and weight of the stainless-steel piece to sink in as you relax. This part is mainly mental . . . the biggest obstacle in this practice.

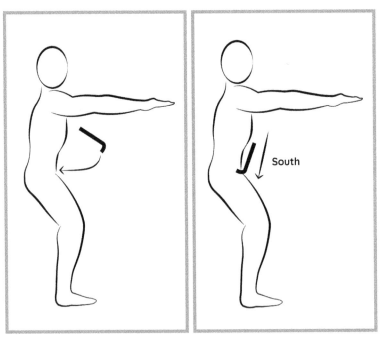

Diagram 60   Diagram 61

6. If you can't find the hole, then with your cock to your belly button, feel for when the base of the sound has reached the base of your perineum. You'll know when because you will be able to feel it there with your other hand on the outside. Keep the tool at the North and gently nudge South into the perineum. *(Diagram 61)*

7. With little tail of the "J" nuzzling into your perineum, lower the long side of the "J" until it is perpendicular to the ground. *(Diagram 62)*

   a. The little tail of the Van Buren sound will naturally enter the bladder's opening and be pointing up to the North *(Diagram 63)*.

   b. The sound is now at the zero point, and you are in.

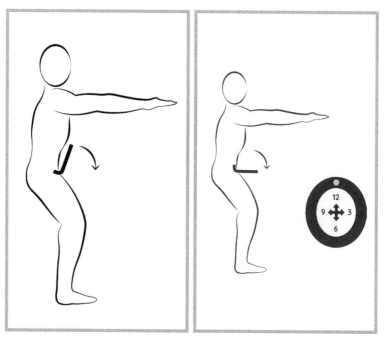

Diagram 62   Diagram 63

EXERCISE 51:

Internal Coordination and De-armoring

1. Where the urethral tube connects to the bladder, it is in the shape of the letter "O."

2. 12 o'clock on the "O" is North.

    a. The 12 o'clock point can be pressed into the by lowering the sound to the perpendicular position with the small tail of the "J" pointing North, and then gently pulling the Van Buren piece away from you.

3. 3 o'clock is reached by pointing the small tail of the "J" to the East; 6 o'clock is South; 9 o'clock is West.

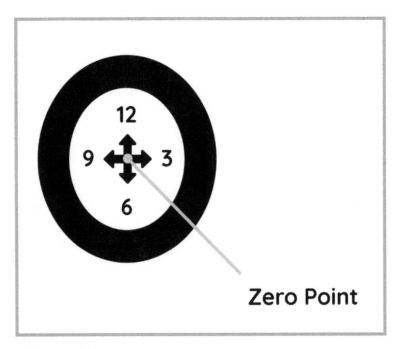

Diagram 64

4. Rotate the sound from 12 o'clock, to 3, to 6, to 9, and back again to 12.

5. Feel into the North, South, East , and West with slight pressure from the different clock posit ions.

6. Be gentle and feel into pressuring along the zero point from the different clock positions. There is a good amount of potential for armoring here at the internal urethral sphincter, inside the bladder.

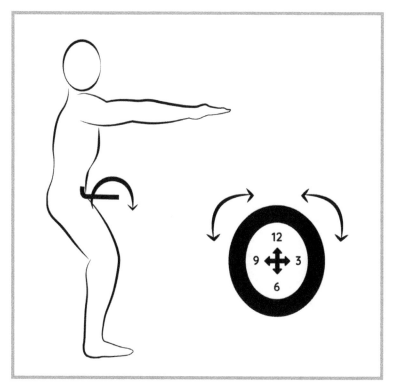

Diagram 65

7. When moving along the zero point away from the body, the sound will place pressure against the pubic bone *(Diagram 66)*. However, exercise caution if moving along the zero point and into the body since the back wall of the bladder does not have the support *(Diagram 67)*.

8. If you want to get the perineum, which is another place where a lot of armoring can build up and likely where most guys get tension before they cum, then with the small tail of the "J" aim down towards the southern position *(Diagram 68)*.

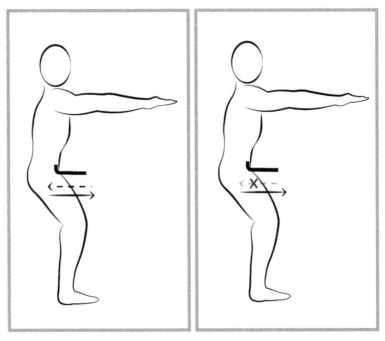

Diagram 66   *Diagram 67*

9. The zero point can be a little more difficult to find with the little tale of the "J" pointing south. Therefore you may wish to first enter the zero point as described before with the tail of the "J" facing up to the North. As you bring the sound to the South of the zero point allow the little tale of the "J" to come out of the bladder's opening and work into the perineum.

10. I usually can find little points of armoring that feels like a needle prick. Hold into the points and keep light pressure along the meridian as you pull the sound out.

11. In other words, if the sound feels armoring somewhere along the urethra, around the opening, or inside the bladder, then move a little behind it, and while keeping gentle pressure with the small tail of the "J" on the same clock position, slowly pull out the sound as you do Exercises 26 and 27, *Genital Breathing* and *Genital Voicing.*

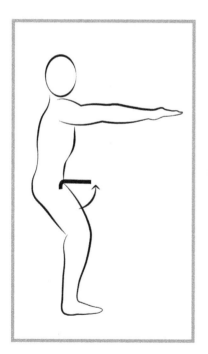

Diagram 68

12. In other words, if the sound is North at 2 o'clock and you feel armoring inside the opening and against the pubic bone, then follow the 2 o'clock meridian as you pull out all the way to the tip of your cock's head.

If you are curious to learn more about fully de-armoring your cock from the inside out, then book a video consultation or purchase the cock de-armoring course by following the link below:

www.aaronmichaelmethod.com/osl_cock_dearmoring

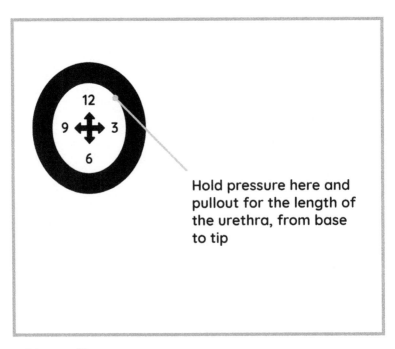

Hold pressure here and pullout for the length of the urethra, from base to tip

Diagram 69

CHAPTER SEVEN:

CHOOSING A PARTNER(S)

DO NOT CAST YOUR PEARLS BEFORE SWINE

Except for breathing, possibly, there is no greater advice you can take to heart than to choose wisely with whom you partner. This I cannot emphasize enough. Not only does the *Optimal Sex Life* have little to do with having sex with aesthetically beautiful partners, it is also much more than the excellent execution of techniques, and the elevated levels of sexual energy you will enjoy. These things can become highly addictive and leave you empty like any other drug. I believe the *Optimal Sex Life* is a coming home to your essence, health, and abundance gifted to you by The Creator. Furthermore, the practice is an important building block and tool for discovering others, pair bonding, long-term relationships and a fruitful family life. I emphasize again that you should choose your partner wisely. If they do not demonstrate the ability or have a track record for handling your heart, their own heart, or the hearts of others with the same care and respect with which one would a child, then they are not ready for the riches which you would open to them sexually from your body, the temple of God.

The exercises in this book are not simply metaphorical practices, but are tied to and work with the anatomy, emotions, psychology, and energy of your body. As much as the experience of optimal sex can become addictive, so, too, can the bonds it creates. An "addiction" to that which is good, balanced, and beneficial to us should be sought out and kept. That which is not should be discarded and avoided. Although not emphasized in this book, ultimately many find these practices to be spiritual and sacred. Whether you do or do not, these exercises should not be taken lightly and practiced with just anybody. Even though approached and celebrated playfully, do not, as is said, cast your pearls before swine, but give whole heartedly to those who cherish you for all you are and who offer themselves in return.

NO ONE IS PERFECT

The summer of 2009 was ending, and I had taken a job at Fitness DK teaching an aerobics class I had come up with by incorporating my past training in fitness and martial arts. It was about six months after my devastating break-up with the girl for whom I had moved to Denmark. Coming out of a rather mournful phase, I had set my mind to finish my MA degree and decided that though I was not looking for a "committed relationship," I was ready to no longer avoid female companionship. I thought a fitness center would be a prime place for meeting women who shared my interest in maintaining one's body, as well as a wonderful place to work while benefiting from a free gym membership. By the time Halloween rolled around, I was casually seeing several women. I was openly honest with them all about this fact. Most said they preferred it this way, as they didn't want to be tied down during their "university experience." For the women who were comfortable with this sort of arrangement, our friendship maintained its sexual spectrum. For the women who seemed to implicate that they would want something more committed, we enjoyed a platonic friendship. This didn't always work out, but that was by far more of the exception than the rule. In fact, the rule in Scandinavia, at the time, seemed to be "have fun" and "keep it cool and casual." Within a short period of time, I had gone from spending the last six months primarily on my own to hanging out with my ever-growing circle of female friends.

The fitness center was throwing a Fall Staff Bash and being a fitness instructor, I was invited. We were all divided into several teams, each dressing up to represent a different region of the world. Fitness instructors, my team, were assigned Africa, and for lack of owning anything else somewhat appropriate, I wore a tam over my then dreadlocks. The receptionist team represented North America, and all wore togas . . . I think in homage to The Statue of Liberty. There was one receptionist who caught my eye. I had briefly introduced myself to her some weeks before and had found her quite attractive. However, at this party and in her toga—really nothing more than a simple sheet—it was her beautiful smile, rich laughter, and the sense of joyfulness that radiated from her that captivated my interest.

At some point well into the night and after the team competitions, we met on the dance floor and had rip-roaring fun shaking our tail feathers. We were speaking intermittently between twirls, dips, smiles, and laughter when she casually asked me, "What do you consider most important in a relationship?" . . . and bang there it was: the million-dollar question I had kicked around in my head for so long, and even more so after the breakup.

Several years prior, my response would have been *honesty*, but I had learned that simply being honest did not always assume responsibility for the bond that easily forms and progresses when intimacy becomes a factor. If this beautiful woman had asked me just before my "failed" yet "learning lesson" of a relationship in Denmark, then I would have answered *honesty and love*, as love (stergos and agape), meant assuming responsibility for one's own and the other's heart. No longer did simple honesty rule, where both parties were individually responsible for their own desires and voicing them. The effect was that I would refrain from sexually engaging with a woman if I could tell that only one of us truly wanted something exclusive, no matter how much to the contrary was "honestly" being spoken, maybe even internally believed—yet clearly signaled in the opposite direction. There was too much room for hurt and pain to turn a blind eye and to allow the other to simply fall in love while remaining ignorant to their true intentions until it became painfully obvious. I felt responsible for those I touched and loved, and had begun to choose the love of friendship over short-lived romances that jeopardized the greater relationship.

However, the answer that came out of my mouth was "Love, Honesty, and Trust." If I had learned anything from my former relationship, then it was that I could be honest with and love until blue in the face, but if there was ultimately no trust in or from the other, then like a house of cards, at the slightest rumor of insecurity, jealousy, or guilt, everything would collapse and come falling right down. Little did I know at the time, but these fundamentals would become the monuments around which she and I would build the foundation for our future relationship. One could even say that they, amongst a few others we have discovered and incorporated along the way, are the cornerstone to our marriage and life together. If I could now emphasize two others, then it would be celebration and responsibility.

My former relationship had love, or at least a strong romance, as well as honesty, but with a family scarred by divorce, my former partner simply could not bring herself to trust me nor to act responsibly with her own or my heart. Her mother had taught her all too well to keep her guard up against men. Almost as a defensive compliment to that advice she would sleep with other men when things were bad between her mom and stepfather. Then, in turn, she would lash out and accuse me of infidelity with any female friends I had. Her jealousy even incorporated my male friends. In fact, it was the closer that she and I became and the more love we shared that then caused her defenses to flare up like gasoline on fire. Romance and honesty simply were not enough. In the end, what we had was undermined by and corroded from a lack of trust and responsibility. What I have discovered with my wife is that no one is perfect or scar-free from their past. Relationships and solid partners are not about perfection, but rather a simple willingness to work together towards overcoming one's own fears, attempting to better oneself individually, and an honest focus to work on your shared relationship, in the spirit of celebrating the mystery of simultaneous union and individuality.

BACKGROUND CHECK

Everyone of course goes through different periods and phases of their life. Be it recent traumatic experiences or simply a bad week, this could cause a person to react in the moment one way or another. We are, after all, human, and affected by our surroundings and timing. However, when feeling into people and assessing whether or not this person might be someone ready, willing, and able to partner, I am looking more at pervasive behavioral patterns. On the one hand, I am wary of resistance, a nearly reflexive resistance, towards love and pair bonding. On the other hand, I am also wary of neediness, either passive or aggressive efforts to dissolve individuality and reshape it into their, your, or some friend's or family member's desired image. Of course, the balance between establishing boundaries and unity can be a bit of a dance. What is important is that you both are capable of navigating these things through open communication, while not reverting into defensiveness, inflexibility, or the unwillingness to hear out the other person. Neither should you allow any other relationships, such as with overbearing mothers, fathers, or friends, to dictate the growth of *your* relationship, nor should you be insensitive, unappreciative or abusive to the circumstances of the other's life.

Consider how potential partners speak of and communicate with or about their parents, siblings, and friends. Do they enjoy the company of their family members? Do they look forward to seeing them? Are they open to introducing you to their family? Does their family enjoy their company? Is the family eager to meet you? Pay attention to whether potential partners make their own decisions or if they are constantly concerned with what their family will think. Are they dependent on their approval? Do they hide or distance themselves from them? Can they speak of their former relationships and sexual encounters? Do they only speak with words of blame and cruelty? Even if hurt, are they free of spite from their last love or lover and able to wish them the best—not out of pity but compassion? Essentially, what we are looking at are attachment behaviors: avoidant, anxious, or secure.

Now these are not to be quick judgments derived from a police-like interrogation. Likely that would only lead to hurt feelings, facile profiling, false conclusions made too quickly, and in general, being deceived by what you already were look-ing for and what is still likely lingering somewhere in your own emotional baggage. Instead, use this sort of information as a means for developing a better understanding of the person with whom you are spending time and have taken an interest in get-ting to know better.

Proceed slowly as if savoring a gourmet course. Be appre-ciative. This is their life they are sharing with you. Bit by bit, bite by succulent bite, and over time you will naturally find the answers to all the questions you want to know as you progress through the initial phases of courtship. This is how it went with my wife. Over walks and meals, we began by get-ting to know one another's interests and sharing stories from our lives. Quite naturally, topics pertaining to friends, fami-ly, and past relationships arose as natural offshoots or segues from stories we imparted, or current interests arising in the moment. Interwoven were our values, dreams, and past scars. We enjoyed each other's company, the process of getting to know one another, and valued the windows we opened into our respective pasts. In fact, the "background check" ques-tions of the previous paragraph were never needed to be asked nor were the answers rushed. Everything simply emerged over time. The flip side of sharing life stories is your reaction to listening to them. Unlike in an interrogation . . . how you feel, as well as the fears or concerns you may have in reaction to the information you receive, should NOT be kept a secret from them. Instead, be considerate of them. Be openhearted and honest.

As previously stated, we are humans. Whether in sharing or listening, we really should not waste time trying to keep up the Wonder Woman or Superman façade. You will only give yourself a headache later when you don't live up to the expectations you set. Not only will your partner see through the pretty picture you have painted, which will birth distrust, but you are actually cheating yourself out of the chance to receive compassion and the opportunity for your partner to give it. Remember *trust*, *love*, and *honesty* . . . celebration and responsibility.

Instead of leading an interrogation, I propose leading by example. Allow yourself to lower your defenses. Openly admit your flaws and that you are not perfect. Take the opportunity to improve and work on them within the support and gusto of a budding relationship. In like fashion, do not use the information and answers you receive from this person to secretly run some form of background check for the purposes of labeling and placing them in a box. Instead, be confident enough to rediscover each other daily, as growth takes time and, therefore, patience. Nevertheless, at the same time do not remain with the goal of changing anyone, but instead only to grow yourself. Even if you could change your partner, it would then set a poor precedent. Ultimately if they are to change, then it is they who must change of their own desire and doing. Furthermore, I AM NOT SUGGESTING IN THE LEAST to be a martyr. Do not waste your time blaming the other person for their faults or wallowing in your own, but instead simply let them know you are not able or willing to grow compatibly with whatever it is that you cannot support . . . be it a partner's history, attitude, habits, or your own issues. Own your inability to support them as a partner without shame or animosity. Bow out with humility, always wishing them the best. As you believe that the problem or solution is not each other, have faith and encouragement that you both will find whatever it is that you need. The universe and future is big, and the potential of the now is truly great.

When you do find the correct partnership, or it finds you, because you're now ready for joy, growth, and grace that is based on trust, love and honesty, and seasoned with celebration and responsibility, INVEST! Invest your heart, your time, and your body. There must be investment if there will ever be growth. At first it will be a bit of a ping-pong back and forth, where your investment rewards the joy they give you and their investment reciprocates the joy you bring them. However, when you both decide to commit to one another, put down all scorecards. Invest with an open and full heart towards your mutually agreed commitment. Do not pretend to be perfect or continue running background checks. Be present. Strive to be the royal, optimal, real, and unique self that you are. Aid and support your partner likewise, and treat them as the King or Queen they are. Then assess you and your partner's growth towards your established goals and commitments. As your goals are achieved, decide together if you wish to set new goals and continue forward. If not, then leave each other better than when you met. If yes, then recommit joyously. Above all else, allow space for transformation. Life is dynamic. Love is centered. Love is tantric, expanding, and extending every-where instrumentally, one fine-tuned note at a time.

If you want to learn more about "Relationship Dynamics and Partner Play," then follow the link and join the email list to stay updated on all future adult sex education courses:

www.aaronmichaelmethod.com/minicourse

ENDNOTES

1. The word choice of "when" elicited a reaction of "yikes" from my editor and rightfully so. However, we chose to stay with the word "when," as opposed to "should," because I find that the sad truth of life is "when"—be it a person, government, or society that is the perpetrator. For these reasons, it is all the more important that we develop our propioception and the ability to act upon it, even if it is simply giving voice to what we feel. Otherwise, how will the world know?

   Wisemen say that rushing is violence
   but so is your silence when it's rooted in compliance
                                   —Rising Appalachia, *Medicine*
                    www.youtube.com/watch?v=czkHmjrFCnM

2. Wayne Elise is the creative director of Charisma Arts, and you can find out more about him at www.charismaarts.com

3. Link to Susanne's website: www.the-gaia-method.com/

4. I included lawyers in my research because I wanted to know if I could legally give these sessions, the risks I would assume, and if so would I be labeled (i.e. file taxes as) a prostitute/sex worker. The answer was not definitive regarding how to file taxes if I began to charge. Prostitution, not pimping/running a brothel, however, is legal in Denmark . . . as long as you pay the state.)

5. Signe V. Bentzen is a therapist with a gift for re-igniting the spark in a marriage, as well as an individual's life. She has also become a phenomenal friend. www.sexologsigne.dk

6. Link to Gry Dagmar's website: www.naervaerd.dk

7. Link to Thomas Meyers' YouTube video "Why Does Massage Hurt": https://www.youtube.com/watch?v=X-G1A-Ct69ug

8. For further details on these practices as well as posture and color visualization exercises for magnified effect, I personally recommend Dr. Saida Désilets' book, *Emergence of the Sensual Woman*, and Mantak Chia's book, *Sexual Reflexology*.

9. By *neotantra* I refer to the modern use of embodied techniques (touch, voice, breath, movements, meditation, etc.) and practices for the purposes of sex and sexuality.

ABOUT
THE AUTHOR

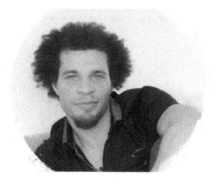

Aaron Michael is a bodyworker and sex coach. He teaches
women, men, and couples how to optimize their sex life for
pleasure and intimacy. He is passionate about providing adults
an avant-garde sex education beyond talk therapy. When he is
not making video courses, writing a book, giving personal sessions, or running international workshops, he enjoys physical
fitness, cooking, and researching new material with his wife . . .
inside and out of the bedroom.

A VERY ABBREVIATED CV:

BA Honors in Linguistics from the University of Michigan
(thesis: *A Linguistic Account of Cult Phenomena*)

Elite MA in Cognitive Semiotics from Aarhus University Denmark (thesis: *An Enactive Approach to Courtship Study: Enactive, Schematic Behavioral Patterns Leading Toward Attachment in Male Initiated Pickup*)

Over 2,000 hours of vaginal de-armoring sessions

Over 250 different women and their partners from diverse ethnic and cultural backgrounds in 1-1 and couples sessions

Assisted and ran workshops in Denmark, Sweden, Tenerife, and the USA.

Featured on Signe Bentzen's former program *Sexperterne* (Denmark's largest newspaper *Ekstra Bladet*)

Interviewed by Julia Bowlin, M.D. (Personal Awareness Medicine), Olivia Bryant (Self-Cervix), Susanne Roursgaard (Gaia Method), Gry Dagmar (NaerVaerd), and Amanda Brown Testa

Collaborates with Susanne Roursgaard, Sanna Sanita, Signe Bentzen, Elma Roura, Gry Dagmar, Krisztina Farkas, Maria Fazzingo , Dr. Hazel-Grace, Dr. Saida Désilets, and several others

ACKNOWLEDGMENTS

Thank you everyone for your unending support to my family and my wife. I was able to focus on writing this book, knowing they had a network of people to love and support them.

Thank you as well for your letters and support. I do not know where to start nor end, for the list would be too long if I were to thank everyone involved in all the small circumstances that made this book possible. From the librarian who gave me some pens, the person who help me print this book, and the one who gave me access to a computer, I want to thank you. This book would not have been born if not for you. I thank you my wife for typing out the entire book and scanning all the drawings. I also thank you all who were so brave to receive sessions in exchange for a testimonial when I was just starting to give sessions. I also want to express my deep gratitude to all those for believing in the importance of this book, taking the time to illustrate, design the cover, and giving me your straightforward opinion. Thank you, Chris Morgan, for your help with the editor. And thank you for the financial help Mogens Sørensen and the man who wished to be unnamed, whose fundings allowed me to hire those whose talents truly turned this book into a work of art. Thank you, Signe Bentzen, for being the first person to suggest that I write a book. Thank you, Susanne Roursgaard, for your encouragement to begin charging money for my sessions and for all the advice in starting a professional career in this field. Thank you, Gry Dagmar Schødt Møberg and Lina Bjørnø, for always reminding me of the importance of getting my work out into the world and into the hands of women and men. Thank you, Domini Dragoone, for your eye for artistic interior design, all the hats you wore in this project, and really turning this work into what I hope to be a masterpiece that will influence the bedrooms and lives of generations to come. Thank you, Adam Beker, for converting my hand illustrations into the needed computer vectors and going way above and beyond the call of what could be expected to get these ever important visuals up to the level of precision needed for readers across the globe to learn and adopt these teachings. Thank you, Nis von Seelen, for working with me to make a cover that still brings me joy. Thank you Filip, Laura, and Elma for your support and encouragement to continue forward and never give up in my time of need. And thank you The One, God, The All, The Universal Love, and the myriad of names failing to capture your oneness for this gift called life and the ability to share it inside and outside of the bedroom and across this planet's green earth, rocky mountains and blue, blue waters.

Lightning Source UK Ltd.
Milton Keynes UK
UKHW021828030820
367624UK00013B/914